NONSTEROIDAL ANTI-INFLAMMATORY DRUGS

Edited by **Ali Gamal Ahmed Al-kaf**

Nonsteroidal Anti-Inflammatory Drugs
http://dx.doi.org/10.5772/65816
Edited by Ali Gamal Ahmed Al-kaf

Contributors

Oya Orun, Pinar Mega Tiber, Sevgi Kocyigit, Raoul Saggini, Ali Al-Kaf, Oliviu Vostinaru, Newman Osafo, Christian Agyare, David Darko Obiri, Aaron Antwi, Giulia Auriemma, Andrea Cerciello, Rita P Aquino, Abdul-Malik Abudunia, Pran Kishore Deb, Raghuprasad Mailabaram, Bilal Al-Jaidi, Mohamed Jamal Saadh

Published by InTech
Janeza Trdine 9, 51000 Rijeka, Croatia

Notice

Publishing Process Manager Nina Kalinic
Technical Editor SPi Global
Cover InTech Design team

First published August, 2017
Printed in Croatia
Legal deposit, Croatia: National and University Library in Zagreb

Additional hard copies can be obtained from orders@intechopen.com

Nonsteroidal Anti-Inflammatory Drugs, Edited by Ali Gamal Ahmed Al-kaf
p. cm.
Print ISBN 978-953-51-3443-5
Online ISBN 978-953-51-3444-2

For EU product safety concerns:
IN TECH d.o.o., Prolaz Marije Krucifikse Kozulić 3, 51000 Rijeka, Croatia,
info@intechopen.com or visit our website at intechopen.com.

Meet the editor

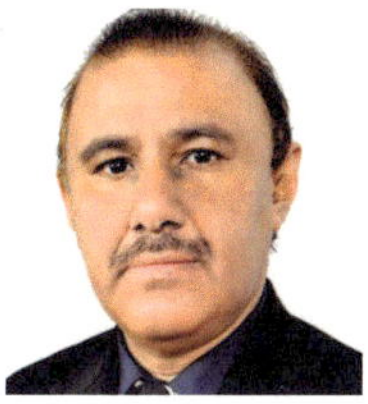

Prof. Al-Kaf has a PhD degree in pharmaceutical sciences from Russia in 2006, and he is a dean of Faculty of Pharmacy at Sana'a University. He is a professor of Medicinal Chemistry Department, a member of many associations and international groups, and an editor and associate editor of some international journals. His interests are synthesis and biological activity of 4-oxo-pyrimidine and quinazolinone-4 derivatives. He studied Yemeni medicinal plants and development and validation of spectrophotometric and HPLC methods for different drugs.
He is an author of more than 40 publications, 4 patents, and 8 books.

Contents

Preface

This book is a unique one in NSAIDs as the whole book consists of many chapters with different topics in the field of NSAIDs, because in medical and pharmaceutical books there is only one chapter that covers the nonsteroidal anti-inflammatory drugs (NSAIDs).

This book intends to provide the reader with a comprehensive overview about the state of the art regarding the use of NSAIDs in physical and rehabilitation medicine and the study of the pharmacodynamics of existing and newly introduced NSAIDs in the management of pain and inflammation. It will also elaborate and refine already known knowledge on the mechanism(s) of nonsteroidal anti-inflammatory agents. This book may provide additional knowledge about the design and development of new drug delivery systems loaded with NSAIDs potentially useful in the treatment of chronic inflammatory–based diseases following circadian cycle, uses of NSAIDs as a source of medicinal plants, and the adverse effects and drug interactions of the nonsteroidal anti-inflammatory drugs

I thank all authors who participate in this book for their valuable, informative, more interested, and important topics in NSAIDs.

The book is a concise form covering all newer drugs that will help the readers to a great extent. The major objective of writing this book is to present the information in a lucid, condensed, and cohesive form, to cater specially the needs of readers in medicine and pharmacy. I also wish to acknowledge indebtedness to all who have assisted with the completion of the book. The cooperation of the publisher, InTech for Science, Technology, and Medicine, is very much appreciated in bringing out this book. The contribution that I received by the sustained cooperation of Ms. Nina Kalinić, Publishing Process Manager, can't be ignored.

Constructive suggestions, comments, and criticism on the subject matter of the book will be gratefully acknowledged, as they will certainly help to improve future editions of the book. It is our hope that this work will prove to be of benefit to students and teachers of pharmacy and science and medical scientists.

Professor Doctor Ali Gamal Al-kaf
Medicinal Chemistry Department
Dean of Faculty of Pharmacy, Sana'a University
Yemen

Chapter 1

Introductory Chapter - The Newest Research in Nonsteroidal Anti-inflammatory Drugs

Ali Gamal Al-kaf

Additional information is available at the end of the chapter

http://dx.doi.org/10.5772/68060

Nonsteroidal anti-inflammatory drugs (NSAIDS) include variety of different agents belonging to different chemical classes. However, many of these agents are carboxylic acids [1]. Most of these drugs have three major effects:

1. Analgesic effect,
2. Antipyretic effect, and
3. Anti-inflammatory effect [1]

The main adverse effects of these drugs are gastric irritation and ulceration, renal damage, and skin reaction [2].

The primary action of these agents is inhibition of cyclooxygenase; the enzyme that catalyses the conversion of arachidonic acid into prostaglandin precursors known as endoperoxides. The resulting decrease in prostaglandin synthesis accounts for most of the actions of those agents [2].

Because of the wide availability and frequency of use of NSAIDs, it is important to be aware of their proper use, dose, and potential side effects. It is difficult to choose the NSAIDs and to predict which is the best one. The response of two identical drugs and doses is clearly different. The most qualified person to help choose and find the optimal NSAID is a health care provider [3].

The aim of writing this book is due to the high importance of NSAIDs, to minimize side effects, to monitor and sensitize the population on the potential adverse effects of misuse, to provide additional knowledge about the design and development of new drug delivery systems loaded with NSAIDs potentially useful in the treatment of chronic inflammatory–based diseases following circadian cycle, and the adverse effects and drug interactions of the non-steroidal anti-inflammatory drugs.

This book covers 14 chapters in which authors from all over the world have participated and includes the following topics:

- Overview of NSAIDs in resource limited countries
- Mechanism of action of nonsteroidal anti-inflammatory drugs
- Nonsteroidal anti-inflammatory drugs on inflammation
- Classification of hypersensitivity reactions to NSAIDs
- Adverse effects and drug interactions of the nonsteroidal anti-inflammatory drugs
- NSAIDs: design and development of innovative oral delivery systems
- Interaction studies of cardiovascular drugs with NSAIDs
- Apoptotic effects of etodolac in breast cancer culture
- Computer aided drug design approaches in the pursuit of the development of selective cyclooxygenase: 2 (COX-2) inhibitor
- Novel drug delivery of nonsteriodal anti-inflammatory drugs (NSAIDs)
- The analgesic and anti-inflammatory effect of terpenoids esters with aminoacids
- Anti-inflammatory and cytotoxicity activity of extract from *Calendula arvensis* flowers
- Analgesics: efficacy and safety of NSAIDs
- Nonsteroidal anti-inflammatory drugs: integrated approach to physical medicine and rehabilitation

This book is a unique one in NSAIDs as a whole book consists of many chapters with different topics in the field of NSAIDs because in medical and pharmaceutical books, there is only one chapter that covers the NSAIDs

I thank all the authors who participated in this book for their valuable, informative, more interested and important topics in NSAIDs.

The book is a concise form covering all newer drugs that will help the readers to a great extent. The major objective of writing this book is to present the information in a lucid, condensed, and cohesive form, to cater specially the needs of readers in medicine and pharmacy. I also wish to acknowledge indebtedness to all who have assisted with the completion of the book. The cooperation of publisher, Intech for Science, Technology and Medicine and publisher is very much appreciated in bringing out this book. The contribution that I received by sustained cooperation of Ms. Nina Kalinić, Publishing Process Manager, cannot be ignored.

http://dx.doi.org/10.5772/68060

Constructive suggestions, comments, and criticism on the subject matter of the book will be delightedly acknowledged, as they will certainly help to improve future editions of the book. It is our hope that this work will prove to be of benefit to the students and teachers of pharmacy, science, and medical scientists.

Author details

Ali Gamal Al-kaf

Address all correspondence to: alialkaf21@gmail.com

Medicinal Chemistry Department, Faculty of Pharmacy, Sana'a University, Yemen

References

[1] RR Nadendla, Principles of Organic Medicinal Chemistry. New Age Publishers, New Delhi, 2005; 322.

[2] KD Tripathi. Essentials of Medical Pharmacology. Seventh edition. Jaypee Brothers Medical Publishers (P) Ltd, New Delhi, 2013; 1020.

[3] https://www.uptodate.com/contents/nonselective-nsaids-overview-of-adverse-effects/abstract/1,2

Chapter 2

Mechanism of Action of Nonsteroidal Anti-Inflammatory Drugs

Newman Osafo, Christian Agyare,
David Darko Obiri and Aaron Opoku Antwi

Additional information is available at the end of the chapter

http://dx.doi.org/10.5772/68090

Abstract

The use of nonsteroidal anti-inflammatory drugs (NSAIDs) dates back to thousands of years when man used natural sources of these agents in a lot of pain and inflammatory conditions. The tone for modern day discovery and use of NSAIDs was set with the discovery of aspirin. Today in addition to aspirin, a host of other NSAIDs of varying potency and efficacy is employed in the management of pain and inflammatory conditions. This chapter looks with key interest in the existing and evolving role of NSAIDs in therapeutics with emphasis on the current insights into their mechanism of action and side effect profiles associated with its use in pain and inflammation as well as its potential therapeutic benefits in cancer chemotherapy.

Keywords: nonsteroidal anti-inflammatory drugs, inflammation, cyclooxygenase, pain, fever

1. Introduction

The history of nonsteroidal anti-inflammatory drugs (NSAIDs) dates as far back as thousands of years with Hippocrates and other physicians prescribing the willow bark for a wide range of conditions [1]. The tone for the modern era of NSAIDs was, however, set by identifying salicin as the willow plant's active ingredient and the subsequent introduction of acetylsalicylic acid by the Bayer Company about two centuries later [2]. Today in addition to aspirin, nonselective NSAIDs, such as piroxicam, mefenamic acid, diclofenac, naproxen, and selective cyclooxygenase-2 (COX-2) inhibiting NSAIDs, such as celecoxib and rofecoxib, remain mainstays of pain and inflammatory disorder therapy.

NSAIDs remain one of the most consumed drugs either by prescription or over-the-counter [3]. Their fever relieving effect has been well documented since their discovery and they have proven effective over the years in controlling pain and inflammatory conditions. It is particularly effective in acute and chronic orthopedic pain (osteoarthritis, ankylosing spondylitis, and rheumatoid arthritis) and postsurgical pain [4]. While these represent the traditional uses of NSAIDs, studies have pointed to their potential in Alzheimer's [5], cancer [6], and Parkinson's disease [7]. Most of these studies exploit the benefits of controlling the underlying inflammatory mechanisms of these diseases.

Nonsteroidal anti-inflammatory drugs (NSAIDs) are a group of therapeutic agents with diverse structural and pharmacodynamics profiles but similar mode of action. Broadly, NSAIDs are grouped into aspirin and nonaspirin NSAIDs. Despite similarities in their mechanism of action and toxicity profiles, they differ slightly in the manner they each interact with the cyclooxygenase enzyme [8]. A more popular classification, however, is based on structural differences and similarities [9]. They are grouped as follows: salicylates (aspirin), aryl alkanoic acids (diclofenac, indomethacin, nabumetone, sulindac), 2-arylpropionic acids or profens (ibuprofen, flurbiprofen, ketoprofen, and naproxen), n-arylanthranilic acids or fenamic acids (mefenamic acids, meclofenamic acid, pyrazolidine derivatives, e.g., phenylbutazone), oxicams (piroxicam, meloxicam), and sulfonamides (nimesulide).

2. Mechanism(s) of NSAIDs action

2.1. COX and COX inhibition

There is overwhelming evidence pointing to the inhibition of cyclooxygenase enzyme as the main mechanism of NSAIDs' analgesic, antipyretic, and anti-inflammatory properties. Since the characterization of this mechanism by Vane for aspirin [10], other drugs in this class have proven consistent this mechanism. This is surprising considering the differences in structures of the individual drugs as described above. Cyclooxygenase (COX) inhibition and the resulting inhibition of prostaglandin and other eicosanoid synthesis mitigate pain, fever, and inflammation. The cyclooxygenase (COX) enzyme also known as prostaglandin endoperoxide H synthase (PGHS) exists in two isoforms: PGHS-1 or COX-1 and PGHS-2 or COX-2. There is a significant structural distinction between the two, with only 60% homology [11]. Although encoded by different genes, both isoforms are membrane-bound glycoproteins that catalyze the formation of prostanoid from arachidonic acid [12].

COX-1 is expressed constitutively in most mammalian cells and tissues such as seminal vesicle, platelets, and endothelium. In quiescent conditions, it performs ongoing regulatory functions referred to as "housekeeping duties." Prostaglandins produced by COX-1 activity perform functions such as gastro and renal protection, macrophage differentiation, platelet aggregation, and mucus production [3, 13]. In inflammatory conditions, molecular studies have demonstrated that COX-1 mRNA and protein expression do not change, confirming their limited role in the inflammatory process [14]. COX-1, however, remains both experimentally and clinically relevant due to the adverse effects triggered by the nonselective inhibition of cyclooxygenase enzymes by some NSAIDs.

COX-2 is an inducible enzyme called upon by tissue injury and other stimuli such as lipopolysaccharide (LPS), interleukin-1, and tumor necrosis factor alpha (TNFα) [15, 16]. It is active at injury sites and in a variety of tissues such as the vascular endothelium, and rheumatoid synovial endothelial cells mediating inflammatory, pain, fever, and carcinogenic responses [17, 18]. A manifold increase in COX-2 levels occurs in inflammatory processes triggering an increased synthesis of pro-inflammatory prostaglandins. Initially thought of as exclusively inducible in nature, studies have shown COX-2 has some constitutive or regulatory roles. Housekeeping duties in reproduction, renal physiology, bone resorption, and neurotransmission have been documented [19, 20].

Indeed studies have shown that both isotypes are constitutive and inducible depending on the physiological conditions [21, 22]. COX-3, a third isotype, has been identified [23]. Its function, distribution, and role in NSAIDs mechanisms are still uncertain and subject of debate [24].

2.2. Pain, fever, and inflammation

The arachidonic acid pathway is central to inflammatory responses and consequently the mechanism of action of NSAIDs. Prostanoids, the end product of this pathway, performs a wide range of physiological functions.

NSAIDs are largely thought of as inhibitors of peripheral pain though several works in literature point to a potential and significant central analgesic activity. At the periphery, a host of mediators occurs to trigger nociception in response to physical, chemical, or electrical stimuli. Prostaglandins act synergistically with other mediators to sensitize nociceptors [10, 25]. Some NSAIDs have exhibited central analgesic effects in several animal models of pain. This is attributed to disruption of synthesis of central prostaglandins and other modulators in the nociceptive pathway. Arguments in favor of central activity stem from studies showing the inhibitory effect of NSAIDs on N-methyl-D-aspartate (NMDA) receptor activation-induced prostaglandin expression in cerebrospinal fluid [26] and antinociceptive effect of spinally administered ibuprofen [27] among others. A classic study by Hunskaar [28] showed overlapping time-effect relationship for aspirin and morphine in the first phase of formalin-induced pain response; a feature highly indicative of central activity.

NSAIDs have proven effective in inflammatory conditions such as arthritis, acute trauma, and pain associated with inflammation. Inflammatory mediators at injury site mediate vasodilation extravasation of protein exudates and nociception. Here, prostaglandins that are key players in this process are inhibited. Though COX inhibition is maintained as the main mechanism for the anti-inflammatory activity of NSAIDs, other mechanisms loosely referred to as non-COX mechanisms have been reported in the literature. NSAIDs are documented to have the suppressive effect in nuclear factor (NF)-κB, a transcription factor for pro-inflammatory proteins such as chemokines, adhesion molecules, and cytokines. NSAIDs also exhibit some suppression of activator protein 1, membrane stabilizing, and inhibition of reactive oxygen species (ROS) production [29–31]. Although these are believed to contribute at a molecular level, it is unclear how they directly aid in the clinical benefits of NSAIDs.

NSAIDs relieve fever by inhibiting COX-mediated prostaglandin synthesis. Upon exposure to external pyrogens, mostly pathogen-associated molecular patterns (lipopolysaccharide, peptidoglycan, viral RNA, etc.), cells of the innate immune system respond by releasing endogenous pyrogens to induce pyrexia. Circulating interleukin-1, interleukin-6, and TNFα gets to the brain and induced the synthesis of prostaglandin via the cyclooxygenase in the preoptic hypothalamic region of the brain. Prostaglandin E_2 (PGE_2) binds to an EP-3 receptor of the endothelium of the hypothalamus to reset the body's thermoregulation. An ensuing physiological process occurs to attain this set temperature. NSAIDs disrupt this process by COX inhibition and therefore have proven useful in curbing the harmful effects of high and persistent temperatures. It is important to note that they have no effect on normal body temperature or atypical rise in temperature such as malignant hyperthermia and heat stroke. Mechanisms in these cases are independent of the COX/prostaglandin inflammatory pathway.

2.3. Structure and mechanisms

Current studies have made it possible to understand the structural basis of both nonselective cyclooxygenase inhibition and COX-2 selective inhibition and the variations in individual NSAID's interactions with COX. The catalytic site of COX-1 is long narrow hydrophobic channel spanning from the membrane-binding domain to the enzyme core. The threshold of the channel is made up of polar groups such as Arg120 and Glu524. NSAIDs bind at the upper portion of this channel specifically at a region near TYR385 and ARG120. Acidic NSAIDs, for instance, interact with ARG120 via hydrophobic and electrostatic forces [32].

While aspirin for instance irreversibly inhibits the COX enzyme by covalently modifying it active Ser529 [10], other NSAIDs such as ibuprofen and naproxen bind reversibly [33]. Studies by Kurumbail et al. [34] revealed a COX-2 3D structure closely resembling COX-1. An extra pocket in the COX-2 catalytic site, however, is created by the valine replacements at positions 523 and 434 (occupied by isoleucine in COX-1). This alteration in structure, among others, is exploited in the design of COX-2 selective drugs.

2.4. H_2S-releasing derivatives of anti-inflammatory drugs

NSAIDs, including selective COX-2 inhibitors, are able to stimulate adherence of leukocytes to the vascular endothelium in the mesenteric circulations [35–38] and that has been strongly associated with NSAID-induced gastric damage [37–39]. With studies pointing to the ability of H_2S donors to suppress leukocyte adherence, it would have been expected that an H_2S-releasing NSAID would not induce leukocyte adherence and will be devoid of the gastric damaging property of NSAIDs. This is actually the case and was realized with studies conducted employing H_2S-releasing derivative of diclofenac (ATB-337) on leukocyte adherence and gastric mucosal integrity in rat [40]. The diclofenac derivative did not stimulate leukocyte adherence and also not elevate lymphocyte function-associated antigen 1 (LFA-1) or intercellular adhesion molecule 1 (ICAM-1), as was observed in diclofenac; also, it did not cause gastric damage [41]. The H_2S-releasing diclofenac, however, did not significantly inhibit gastric prostaglandin synthesis and systemic COX-1 activity [40]. Similar profile in activity was also observed in the H_2S-releasing derivative of indomethacin (ATB-343).

H_2S-releasing derivatives of NSAIDs have also been established to reduce infiltration of leukocytes in models of inflammation. A diclofenac derivative has been shown to reduce

LPS-induced infiltration of neutrophils into the lung and liver [41]; also an H_2S-releasing derivative of mesalamine profoundly reduced granulocyte infiltration in a mouse model of colitis [42] with effect significantly greater than that observed in the parent molecules in each case. H_2S-releasing diclofenac was also realized to be more potent than diclofenac in reducing paw edema in the carrageenan-induced paw edema model in rat.

The upregulation in TNF-α and COX-2 expression in the rat stomach [43, 44] by NSAIDs is not observed in the H_2S-releasing derivatives of NSAIDs despite their ability to cause marked suppression of gastric prostaglandin synthesis [40]. Moreover, these derivatives inhibit endotoxin-induced NF-κB activation and the associated increase in plasma TNF-α, nitrate, and nitrite [41].

2.5. Antitumor action of NSAIDs

NSAIDs have many effects that might contribute to chemoprevention of cancers such as colorectal cancer (CRC). This mode of prevention can be either COX-dependent or COX-independent which can be synergistic at different steps of this multistep process [45] with evidence for replacement of adenomatous polyposis coli (APC) function by NSAIDs. In this direction, sulindac and indomethacin have been shown to inhibit tumorigenesis through inhibition of peroxisome proliferator-activated receptor delta (PPARδ), a gene that is normally regulated by APC [46]. Currently, alterations of the COX-2-related pathways are in primary focus [47].

With NSAIDs being transcriptional inhibitors of COX-2 expression [48], these agents might selectively inhibit the induction of apoptosis in human intestinal stem cells with aberrant Wnt signaling [49]. The most compelling evidence of the possible chemopreventive action of some NSAIDs was the finding that aspirin reduces the risk of CRC in individuals with elevated COX-2 expression but not in those without [50] with associated reduced mortality [51], in an observational study. This was however experimentally confirmed when data affirmed the involvement of prostaglandins and nonprostaglandin COX-2 products were central to the development of CRC [52].

Measurable levels of NSAID-activated gene-1 (NAG-1) were detected in an NSAID-treated human CRC cell line. NAG-1 belongs to the transforming growth factor beta (TGFβ)-superfamily of growth factors and plays a significant role in apoptosis and tumorigenesis. In the CRC cells, NAG-1 expression positively correlates apoptosis and inversely correlates with COX-2 expression, with NAG-1 upregulation linked with NSAID administration in a Prostaglandin-independent manner [53]. Overexpression of NAG-1 in APC-mutated Min/+ mice results in reduced tumorigenesis. Interestingly, however, high COX-2 expression in colorectal tumors is associated with decreased expression of NAG-1, suggesting a reciprocal relationship [54]. It is henceforth being speculated that high levels of COX-2 in colorectal tumors suppress the expression of NAG-1; hence induction of NAG-1 by NSAIDs might contribute to the chemopreventive action of these agents [55].

Aspirin has a unique property of acetylating COX-2, which is not seen in other NSAIDs. This switches COX-2 from synthesizing prostaglandins (PGE_2) (tumor promotion) to antitumorigenic 15-epi-lipoxin-A_4 (LXA_4), a 5-lipoxygenase catalyzed reaction. 15-epi-lipoxin-A_4 is anti-inflammatory as well as anti-proliferative on carcinoma cells [56]. This effect of aspirin is seen at low antiplatelet doses with one study with 75 mg/day for 10 days not only reducing PGE_2 formation and white cell accumulation in inflamed tissues but also significantly increasing local lipoxin production [57]. This establishes that the anticancer potential of aspirin may be due to lipoxin production.

Several studies also point to COX-2 independent actions may also play a role in apoptosis and such pathways have been realized to be sensitive to NSAIDs. Not all human CRCs express COX-2 and produce prostaglandins [58, 59]. However, the potency of NSAIDs to inhibit proliferation is similar to COX-2 producing CRC [60]. This is suggestive of the fact that the antitumor actions of NSAIDs are not necessarily via inhibition of COX-2 or prostaglandin formation [45, 59]. Sulindac reduces the number of aberrant crypt foci and adenomas in patients under conditions when etodolac, COX-2 inhibitor, was ineffective [61]. Moreover, sulindac was also found to significantly increase NAG-1 even in COX-2-deficient tumor cell lines [53].

The potential COX-2-independent mechanism of NSAIDs' antineoplastic action includes downregulation of proto-oncogenes, such as *c-myc*, and transcriptional factors such as PPARδ, NF-κB, prostate apoptosis response-4 (PAR-4), and *Bcl-2*. The most recent therapeutic approach therefore entails combining NSAIDs and epidermal growth factor (EGF) receptor inhibitors in chemoprevention of CRC [62].

3. Conclusion

The therapeutic importance of NSAIDs in the management of acute and chronic pain and inflammation cannot be overemphasized. Also with the emergence of their therapeutic benefits in cancers, it is worth chronicling its pharmacological profile, specifically their established and expected mechanistic pathways of eliciting their activity. With promising outcomes in the experimental studies with improved gastrointestinal effects associated with modified NSAIDs and potential anticancer activity of NSAIDs, we strongly believe there is more to NSAIDs than we currently know. This chapter will henceforth give an insight into what is known and what could be possibly done in advancing the therapeutic potentials of NSAIDs beyond the management of pain and inflammation as we know.

Author details

Newman Osafo[1]*, Christian Agyare[2], David Darko Obiri[1] and Aaron Opoku Antwi[1]

*Address all correspondence to: nosafo.pharm@knust.edu.gh

1 Department of Pharmacology, Kwame Nkrumah University of Science and Technology, Kumasi, Ghana

2 Department of Pharmaceutics, Kwame Nkrumah University of Science and Technology, Kumasi, Ghana

References

[1] Rao P, Knaus EE. Evolution of nonsteroidal anti-inflammatory drugs (NSAIDs): Cyclooxygenase (COX) inhibition and beyond. Journal of Pharmacy & Pharmaceutical Sciences. 2008;**11**(2):81-110

[2] Vane JR. The fight against rheumatism: From willow bark to COX-1 sparing drugs. Journal of Physiology and Pharmacology. 2000;**51**:573-586

[3] Bozimowski G. A review of nonsteroidal anti-inflammatory drugs. AANA Journal. 2015;**83**(6):425-433

[4] KuKanich B, Bidgood T, Knesl O. Clinical pharmacology of nonsteroidal anti-inflammatory drugs in dogs. Veterinary Anaesthesia and Analgesia. 2012;**39**:69-90

[5] Etminan M, Gill S, Samii A. Effect of non-steroidal anti-inflammatory drugs on risk of Alzheimer's disease: Systematic review and meta-analysis of observational studies. British Medical Journal. 2003;**327**:128-132

[6] Zhu JX, Song XQ, Lin HP, Young DC, Yan SQ, Marquez VE, Chen CS. Using cyclooxygenase-2 inhibitors as molecular platforms to develop a new class of apoptosis inducing agents. Journal of the National Cancer Institute. 2002;**95**:1745-1757

[7] Teismann P, Tieu K, Choi DK, Wu DC, Naini A, Hunot S, Vila M, Jackson-Lewis V, Przedborski S. Cyclooxygenase-2 is instrumental in Parkinson's disease neuro-degeneration. Proceedings of the National Academy of Sciences of the United States of America. 2003;**100**:5473-5478

[8] Vonkeman HE, van de Laar MA. Nonsteroidal anti-inflammatory drugs: Adverse effects and their prevention. Seminars in Arthritis and Rheumatism. 2010;**39**:294-312

[9] Meek IL, van de Laar MAFJ, Vonkeman HE. Non-steroidal anti-inflammatory drugs: An overview of cardiovascular risks. Pharmaceuticals (Basel). 2010;**3**(7):2146-2162

[10] Vane JR. Inhibition of prostaglandin synthesis as a mechanism of action for aspirin-like drugs. Nature New Biology. 1971;**231**:232-235

[11] Jones DA, Carlton DP, McIntyre TM, Zimmerman GA, Prescott SM. Molecular cloning of human prostaglandin endoperoxide synthase type II and demonstration of expression in response to cytokines. The Journal of Biological Chemistry. 1993;**268**:9049-9054

[12] Liu J. Non-steroidal anti-inflammatory drugs and cancer, with an especial focus on esophageal cancer. Asian Pacific Journal of Cancer Prevention. 2011;**12**:3159-3168

[13] Coleman RA, Smith WL, Narimiya S. Classification of prostanoid receptors: Properties, distribution and structure of the receptors and their subtypes. Pharmacological Reviews. 1994;**46**:205-229

[14] Smith CJ, Zhang Y, Koboldt CM, Muhammad J, Zweifel BS, Shaffer A, Talley JJ, Masferrer JL, Seibert K, Isakson PC. Pharmacological analysis ofcyclooxygenase-1 in

inflammation. Proceedings of the National Academy of Sciences of the United States of America. 1998;**95**:13313-13318

[15] Masferrer JL, Isakson PC, Seibert K. Cyclooxygenase-2 inhibitors: A new class of anti-inflammatory agents that spare the gastrointestinal tract. Gastroenterology Clinics of North America. 1996;**25**:363-72

[16] Meade EA, Smith WL, DeWitt DL. Differential inhibition of prostaglandin endoperoxide synthase (cyclooxygenase) isozymes by aspirin and other non-steroidal anti-inflammatory drugs. The Journal of Biological Chemistry. 1993;**268**:6610-6614

[17] Atkinson TJ, Fudin J, Jahn HL, Kubotera N, Rennick AL, Rhorer M. What's new in NSAID pharmacotherapy: Oral agents to injectables. Pain Medicine. 2013;**14**(1):11-17

[18] Haeggström JZ, Rinaldo-Matthis A, Wheelock CE, Wetterholm A. Advances in eicosanoid research, novel therapeutic implications. Biochemical and Biophysical Research Communications. 2010;**396**(1):135-139

[19] Breder CD, DeWitt DL, Kraig RP. Characterization of inducible cyclooxygenase in rat brain. Journal of Comparative Neurology. 1995;**355**:296-315

[20] Pilbeam CC, Fall PM, Alander CB, Raisz LG. Differential effects of nonsteroidal antiinflammatory drugs on constitutive and inducible prostaglandin G/H synthase in cultured bone cells. Journal of Bone and Mineral Research. 1997;**12**:1198-1203

[21] Wooten JG, Blikslager AT, Ryan KA, et al. Cyclooxygenase expression and prostanoid production in pyloric and duodenal mucosae in dogs after administration of nonsteroidal anti-inflammatory drugs. American Journal of Veterinary Research. 2008;**69**:457-464

[22] Lascelles BD, King S, Roe S, et al. Expression and activity of COX-1 and 2 and 5-LOX in joint tissues from dogs with naturally occurring coxofemoral joint osteoarthritis. Journal of Orthopaedic Research. 2009;**27**:1204-1208

[23] Chandrasekharan NV, Dai H, Roos KL, Evanson NK, Tomsik J, Elton TS, Simmons DL. COX-3, a cyclooxygenase-1 variant inhibited by acetaminophen and other analgesic/antipyretic drugs: Cloning, structure and expression. Proceedings of the National Academy of Sciences. 2002;**99**:13926-13931

[24] Kis B, Snipes JA, Busija DW. Acetaminophen and the cyclooxygenase-3 puzzle: Sorting out facts, fictions, and uncertainties. Journal of Pharmacology and Experimental Therapeutics . 2005;**315**:1-7

[25] Ferreira SH, Moncada S, Vane JR. Indomethacin and aspirin abolish prostaglandin release from spleen. Nature. 1971; **231**:237-9

[26] Bjorkman R. Central antinociceptive effects of non-steroidal anti-inflammatory drugs and paracetamol. Acta Anaesthesiologica Scandinavica. 1995;**39**(103):1-44

[27] Wang BC, Li D, Hiller J. The antinociceptive effect of S-(+) ibuprofenin rabbits: Epidural versus intravenous administration. Anesthesia & Analgesia . 1995;**80**:92-96

[28] Hunskaar S. Similar effects of acetylsalicylic acid and morphine on immediate responses to acute noxious stimulation. Pharmacology & Toxicology. 1987;**60**:167-170

[29] Tegeder I, Niederberger E, Israr E, Gühring H, Brune K, Euchenhofer C, Grösch S, Geisslinger G. Inhibition of NF-kappa B and AP-1 activation by R- and S-flurbiprofen. The FASEB Journal. 2001;**15**:595-597

[30] Bryant CE, Farnfield BA, Janicke HJ. Evaluation of the ability of carprofen and flunixin meglumine to inhibit activation of nuclear factor kappa B. American Journal of Veterinary Research. 2003;**64**:211-215

[31] Mounnissamy VM, Kavimani S, Balu V, Drlin QS. Evaluation of anti-inflammatory and membrane stabilizing properties of ethanol extract of *Canjera rehedi*. Iranian Journal of Pharmacology & Therapeutics. 2008;**6**:235-237

[32] Mancini JA, Riendeau D, Falgueyret JP, Vickers PJ, O'Neill GP. Arginine 120 of prostaglandin G/H synthase-1 is required for the inhibition by nonsteroidal anti-inflammatory drugs containing a carboxylic acid moiety. The Journal of Biological Chemistry. 1995;**270**:29372-29377

[33] Stanford N, Roth GJ, Shen TY, Majerus PW. Lack of covalent modification of prostaglandin synthetase (cyclo-oxygenase) by indomethacin. Prostaglandins. 1977;**13**:669-675

[34] Kurumbail R, Stevens A, Gierse J, McDonald J, Stegeman RA, Pak JY, Gildehaus D, Miyashiro JM, Penning TD, Seibert K, Isakson PC, Stallings WC. Structural basis for selective inhibition of cyclooxygenase-2 by anti-inflammatory agents. Nature. 1996;**384**:644-648

[35] Asako H, Kubes P, Wallace J, Gaginella T, Wolf RE, Granger DN. Indomethacin-induced leukocyte adhesion in mesenteric venules: Role of lipoxygenase products. American Journal of Physiology. 1992;**262**:G903-G908

[36] Asako H, Kubes P, Wallace J, Wolf RE, Granger DN. Modulation of leukocyte adhesion to rat mesenteric venules by aspirin and salicylate. Gastroenterology. 1992;**103**(1):146-152

[37] Wallace JL, McKnight W, Miyasaka M, Tamatani T, Paulson J, Anderson DC, Granger DN, Kubes P. Role of endothelial adhesion molecules in NSAID-induced gastric mucosal injury. American Journal of Physiology. 1993;**265**:G993-G998

[38] Wallace JL, McKnight W, Reuter BK, Vergnolle N. NSAID-induced gastric damage in rats: Requirement for inhibition of both cyclooxygenase 1 and 2. Gastroenterology. 2000;**119**:706-714

[39] Wallace JL, Arfors KE, McKnight GW. A monoclonal antibody against the CD18 leukocyte adhesion molecule prevents indomethacin-induced gastric damage in the rabbit. Gastroenterology. 1991;**100**:878-883

[40] Wallace JL, Caliendo G, Santagada V, Cirino G, Fiorucci S. Gastrointestinal safety and anti-inflammatory effects of a hydrogen sulfide-releasing diclofenac derivative in the rat. Gastroenterology. 2007;**132**:261-271

[41] Li L, Rossoni G, Sparatore A, Lee LC, Del Soldato P, Moore PK. Anti-inflammatory and gastrointestinal effects of a novel diclofenac derivative. Free Radical Biology and Medicine. 2007;**42**:706-719

[42] Fiorucci S, Orlandi S, Mencarelli A, Caliendo G, Santagada V, Distrutti E, Santucci L, Cirino G, Wallace JL. Enhanced activity of a hydrogen sulphide-releasing derivative of mesalamine (ATB-429) in a mouse model of colitis. British Journal of Pharmacology. 2007;**150**:996-1002

[43] Fiorucci S, Antonelli E, Distrutti E, Rizzo G, Mencarelli A, Orlandi S, Zanardo R, Renga B, Di Sante M, Morelli A, Cirino G, Wallace JL. Inhibition of hydrogen sulfide generation contributes to gastric injury caused by anti-inflammatory nonsteroidal drugs. Gastroenterology. 2005;**129**:1210-1224

[44] Davies NM, Sharkey KA, Asfaha S, Macnaughton WK, Wallace JL. Aspirin induces a rapid up-regulation of cyclooxygenase-2 in the rat stomach. Alimentary Pharmacology & Therapeutics. 1977;**11**:1101-1108

[45] Rigas B, Shiff SJ. Nonsteroidal anti-inflammatory drugs and the induction of apoptosis in colon cells: Evidence for PHS-dependent and PHS-independent mechanisms. Apoptosis. 1999;**4**(5):373-381

[46] He TC, Chan TA, Vogelstein B, Kinzler KW. PPAR delta is an APC-regulated target of nonsteroidal anti-inflammatory drugs. Cell. 1999;**99**(3):335-345

[47] Wang D, Dubois RN. The role of COX-2 in intestinal inflammation and colorectal cancer. Oncogene. 2010;**29**(6):781-788

[48] Wu KK. Salicylates and their spectrum of activities. Anti-Inflammatory, Anti-Allergy Agents in Medicinal Chemistry. 2007;**6**:278-292

[49] Qiu W, Wang X, Leibowitz B, Liu H, Barker N, Okada H, et al. Chemoprevention by non-steroidal anti-inflammatory drugs eliminates oncogenic intestinal stem cells via SMAC-dependent apoptosis. Proceedings of the National Academy of Sciences of the United States of America. 2010;**107**(46):20027-20032

[50] Chan AT, Ogino S, Fuchs CS. Aspirin and the risk of colorectal cancer in relation to the expression of COX-2. The New England Journal of Medicine. 2007;**356**(21):2131-2142

[51] Chan AT, Ogino S, Fuchs CS. Aspirin use and survival after diagnosis of colorectal cancer. Journal of the American Medical Association. 2009;**302**(6):649-658

[52] Fischer SM, Hawk E, Lubet RA. Non-steroidal anti-inflammatory drugs and coxibs in chemoprevention: A commentary based primarily on animal studies. Cancer Prevention Research. 2011;**4**(11):1728-1735

[53] Baek SJ, Kim KS, Nixon JB, Wilson LC, Eling TE. Cyclooxygenase inhibitors regulate the expression of a TGF-beta superfamily member that has proapoptotic and antitumorigenic activities. Molecular Pharmacology. 2001;**59**(4):901-908

[54] Iguchi G, Chrysovergis K, Lee SH, Baek SJ, Langenbach R, Eling TE. A reciprocal relationship exists between non-steroidal anti-inflammatory drug-activated gene-1 (NAG-1) and cyclooxygenase-2. Cancer Letters. 2009;**282**(2):152-158

[55] Schrör K. Pharmacology and cellular/molecular mechanisms of action of aspirin and non-aspirin NSAIDs in colorectal cancer. Best Practice & Research Clinical Gastroenterology. 2011;**25**:473-484

[56] Claria J, Lee MH, Serhan CN. Aspirin-triggered lipoxins (15-epi-LX) are generated by the human lung adenocarcinoma cell line (A549)-neutrophil interactions and are potent inhibitors of cell proliferation. Molecular Medicine. 1996;**2**(5):583-596

[57] Morris T, Stables M, Hobbs A, de Souza P, Colville-Nash P, Warner T, et al. Effects of low-dose aspirin on acute inflammatory responses in humans. The Journal of Immunology. 2009;**183**(3):2089-2096

[58] Marnett LJ. Aspirin and the potential role of prostaglandins in colon cancer. Cancer Research. 1992;**52**(20):5575-5589

[59] Hanif R, Pittas A, Feng Y, Koutsos MI, Qiao L, Staiano-Coico L, Shiff SI, Rigas B. Effects of nonsteroidal anti-inflammatory drugs on proliferation and on induction of apoptosis in colon cancer cells by a prostaglandin-independent pathway. Biochemical Pharmacology. 1996;**52**(2):237-245

[60] Dihlmann S, Siermann A, von Knebel Doeberitz M. The nonsteroidal anti-inflammatory drugs aspirin and indomethacin attenuate beta-catenin/TCF-4 signaling. Oncogene. 2001;**20**(5):645-653

[61] Takayama T, Nagashima H, Maeda M, Nojiri S, Hirayama M, Nakano Y, et al. Randomized double-blind trial of sulindac and etodolac to eradicate aberrant crypt foci and to prevent sporadic colorectal polyps. Clinical Cancer Research. 2011;**17**(11):3803-3811

[62] Torrance CJ, Jackson PE, Montgomery E, Kinzler KW, Vogelstein B, Wissner A, Nunes M, Frost P, Discafani CM. Combinatorial chemoprevention of intestinal neoplasia. Nature Medicine. 2000;**6**:1024-1028

Chapter 3

Adverse Effects and Drug Interactions of the Non-Steroidal Anti-Inflammatory Drugs

Oliviu Vostinaru

Additional information is available at the end of the chapter

http://dx.doi.org/10.5772/intechopen.68198

Abstract

The aim of this chapter is to increase the awareness of health-care professionals concerning potential adverse effects and drug interactions of non-steroidal anti-inflammatory drugs (NSAIDs), which are among the most widely prescribed medicines, globally. They have a variety of clinical applications due to their anti-inflammatory, analgesic, antipyretic, or antithrombotic effect, but these drugs are not entirely innocuous, since they could increase the risk of gastrointestinal and cardiovascular complications. Furthermore, the drugs from this class have the potential of altering the pharmacokinetics of associated drugs, and also pharmacodynamic interactions have been reported. The clinical significance, mechanisms, and epidemiology of the adverse effects and drug interactions of NSAIDs are presented in this chapter. Prevention strategies for particularly high-risk groups of patients are also exposed. Detailed and up-to-date information regarding the adverse effects and drug interactions of NSAIDs are needed for all healthcare professionals in order to maximize efficacy in treating various illnesses while minimizing the risks for the patients.

Keywords: NSAIDs, gastrointestinal, cardiovascular adverse effects, nephropathy, hepatotoxicity, drug interactions

1. Introduction

The non-steroidal anti-inflammatory drugs (NSAIDs) are among the most successful medicines in the world, being used by large numbers of patients, due to their anti-inflammatory, analgesic, and antipyretic effects. Since the discovery of acetylsalicylic acid (aspirin) in the nineteenth century by F. Hoffmann, more than 50 different molecules have been marketed worldwide. NSAIDs are usually prescribed in chronic inflammatory conditions, but they are also extensively used as over-the-counter (OTC) drugs in a variety of inflammatory processes, mild-to-moderate pain or fever. Other clinical uses (e.g. low-dose aspirin for cardioprotection) are also very popular.

Chemically, NSAIDs are extremely heterogeneous: salicylic acid derivatives (aspirin, diflunisal), indoles (indomethacin), fenamic acid derivatives (mefenamic acid, meclofenamic acid), acetic acid derivatives (diclofenac, ketorolac), propionic acid derivatives (ibuprofen, ketoprofen, naproxen), enolic acid derivatives (piroxicam, meloxicam), or diaryl heterocyclic compounds (celecoxib, etoricoxib) [1]. Most of the NSAIDs are organic acids, with low pKa values, capable of accumulation in the inflamed tissues, characterized by acidic pH.

Pharmacologically, all NSAIDs share a common mechanism of action, discovered by J.R. Vane in 1971: they act as competitive and reversible inhibitors of Prostaglandin G/H synthase (also known as cyclooxygenase or COX), thus reducing the formation of various prostaglandins [2]. The only exception is acetylsalicylic acid (aspirin), which irreversibly acetylates a key amino acid (serine 529) situated in the active site of COX-1, with the formation of a covalent bond, which leads to permanent enzyme inhibition. A series of studies characterized at least two isoforms of COX in humans:

- COX-1, a constitutive enzyme, normally expressed in many cells, which generates prostaglandins directly involved not only in the protection of gastric mucosa but also in platelet and renal homeostasis. The inhibition of this isoform is considered to be responsible for the gastric adverse effects of non-selective NSAIDs.
- COX-2, induced by pro-inflammatory cytokines or aggression of the tissues, which generates prostaglandins involved in pain, fever, and inflammation. Also, COX-2 can be responsible for some physiological functions.

Depending on the relative selectivity for COX isoforms, two types of NSAIDs have been developed:

- Non-selective (traditional) NSAIDs (ibuprofen, diclofenac, indomethacin, etc.), which inhibit both isoforms of COX, with high potential of inducing gastric irritation.
- COX-2 selective drugs (coxibs, nimesulide, meloxicam), which selectively inhibit COX-2, better tolerated by the gastric mucosa, but with different safety issues.

A key feature of NSAID class is that, partially, both beneficial and adverse effects are caused by the same mechanism of action: inhibition of prostaglandin biosynthesis [1, 3].

2. Adverse effects of NSAIDs

The adverse drug reactions (ADRs) are a major health issue worldwide, causing frequent hospital admissions and being one of the leading causes of mortality [4]. Although adverse effects of non-steroidal anti-inflammatory drugs (NSAIDs) affect a limited percentage of users, the widespread use of these medicines can cause significant health problems. The probability of suffering severe adverse effects is correlated with the dose and the age of the patients, the elderly being more vulnerable. Lower starting doses and reduction of doses in patients at risk are good preventive strategies, but further studies are necessary in order to develop genetic or biochemical markers of NSAID toxicity, in order to better anticipate the advent of an unwanted drug-induced adverse effect [5].

The adverse effects of NSAIDs can be manifested at different levels.

2.1. Gastrointestinal

The gastrointestinal (GI) adverse effects of NSAIDs are considered to be a hallmark of this pharmacological class, affecting 10–60% of patients [6]. They can include an array of symptoms and manifestations varying in severity from simple dyspepsia with pyrosis to fully developed gastric or intestinal ulcer. The ulcerations can become complicated with acute bleeding and perforation, a life-threatening situation. The most frequent adverse effects of NSAIDs at gastrointestinal level together with the additional risk factors are presented in **Table 1**.

The propensity of NSAIDs to induce gastrointestinal adverse effects depends on the molecule and mode of action. The non-selective NSAIDs frequently cause gastrointestinal damage, while the COX-2 selective NSAIDs have a dramatically improved gastric tolerability. The mechanism of NSAID-induced gastrointestinal damage has been extensively studied [5, 6].

The non-selective NSAIDs can induce lesions of the gastrointestinal mucosa by a topical erosive effect combined with a systemic effect characterized by depletion of prostaglandins synthesized by COX-1 (**Figure 1**). Normally, these "good" prostanoids stimulate the synthesis and secretion of mucus and bicarbonate, increase the blood flow, and promote epithelial proliferation. By removing these beneficial effects, non-selective NSAIDs create a gastric environment more susceptible to topical erosion by exogenous and endogenous factors. Thus, the acidic properties of most NSAIDs initiate mucosal damage because the drug molecules remain in a non-ionized lipophilic form in the acid environment of the stomach, entering into surface epithelial cells where they dissociate, trapping hydrogen ions and inducing lesions. The NSAID molecules additionally reduce the hydrophobicity of gastric mucus, allowing the hydrochloric acid and pepsin to attack the surface epithelium [5, 6].

Also, the decrease of TXA2, process which can subsequently favor bleeding, is an additional mechanism of NSAID-induced gastric damage.

Affected organ system	Symptoms and manifestations	Additional risk factors
Gastrointestinal tract	Dyspepsia with pyrosis, Abdominal pain, Nausea, Anorexia, Gastric erosions, Ulcers, Perforation, Gastrointestinal hemorrhage, Anemia	History of GI ulcer, *Helicobacter pylori*, Age above 60, High doses of NSAIDs, Use of anticoagulants and corticosteroids, Use of multiple NSAIDs

Adapted from Refs. [1, 6].

Table 1. Adverse effects of NSAIDs at gastrointestinal level and additional risk factors.

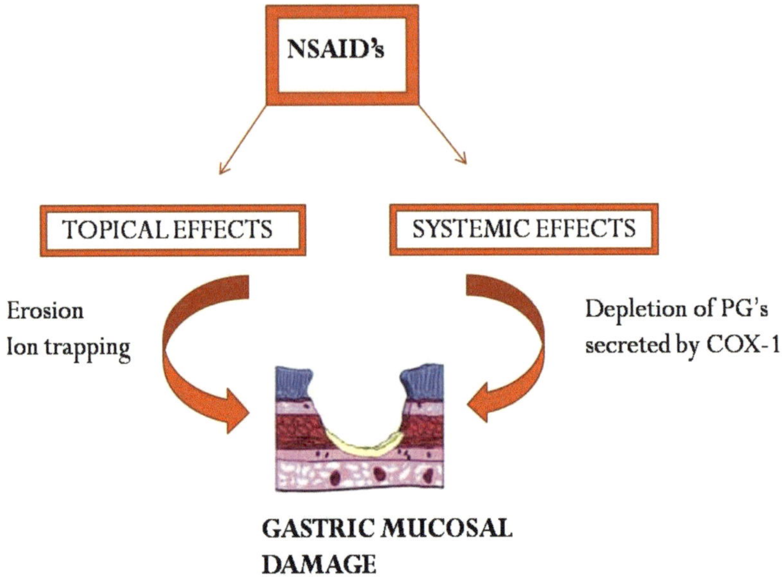

Figure 1. Mechanisms of NSAID-induced gastrointestinal damage.

Whether the direct, topical erosive effect of non-selective NSAIDs or the systemic depletion of "good" prostaglandins is the key factor responsible for the apparition of gastrointestinal damage, is still a matter of controversy.

Several large-scale epidemiological studies have been performed to gather valuable information regarding the gastrointestinal (GI) safety profile of the NSAID class.

For the non-selective NSAIDs, the Arthritis, Rheumatism, and Ageing Medical Information Systems (ARAMIS) study reported that the rate of gastrointestinal events was six times higher in patients taking NSAIDs than in non-users [7]. The meta-analysis of Gabriel et al. indicated that the relative risk (RR) of the first gastrointestinal event is 2.4 (CI 95%: 2.2–2.7) but becomes 4.8 (CI 95%: 4.0–5.6) if a previous history of ulcer exists [8]. Also, another study identified that the relative risk for adverse GI events increased with age, from 1.8 in younger patients to 3.5 in patients between 60 and 75 years old [9].

Furthermore, the Paracetamol, Aspirin, and Ibuprofen New Tolerability (PAIN) study demonstrated that ibuprofen (<1200 mg/day) was similar to acetaminophen (<3000 mg/day) in terms of the incidence of significant GI adverse effects and that statistically significant fewer events were associated with ibuprofen in comparison with aspirin (<3000 mg/day) during 1–7 days of treatment [10].

For the COX-2 selective NSAIDs, the Celecoxib Long-Term Arthritis Safety Study (CLASS) trial randomized patients with rheumatoid arthritis to either celecoxib 400 mg twice daily, ibuprofen 800 mg three times daily, or diclofenac 75 mg twice daily. After 6 months, significantly lower GI events were seen in celecoxib group (RR 0.59; 95% CI: 0.38–0.94) [11].

For etoricoxib, gastrointestinal adverse events were evaluated by combined analysis of 10 clinical trials enrolling 3142 patients. According to this study, etoricoxib halves both perforation and confirmed and unconfirmed bleeding, compared to non-selective NSAIDs [12].

Finally, a meta-analysis of 112 large-scale randomized clinical trials revealed that the risk of ulcer and serious GI complications associated with coxibs were lower than non-selective NSAIDs (RR 0.49; 95% CI: 0.38–0.62 vs. RR 0.55; 95% CI: 0.38–0.80) [13].

The management of patients receiving NSAIDs regarding gastrointestinal toxicity should take into consideration several key facts [5, 14]:

- The lowest dose should be used for the shortest period of time.
- Simultaneous administration of anticoagulants and corticosteroids should be avoided.
- *Helicobacter pylori* infection should be eradicated if present.
- NSAIDs with high GI toxicity (piroxicam, ketoprofen, ketorolac) should be avoided.
- The gastric damage can be reduced by associating NSAIDs with misoprostol or proton pump inhibitors (PPIs).
- If no gastrointestinal risk factors are present, non-selective NSAIDs are preferred.
- If one or more GI risk factors are present, coxibs should be used or non-selective NSAIDS + proton pump inhibitors (PPIs).

2.2. Cardiovascular

Based on currently available data, regulatory agencies from EU (EMEA) and USA (FDA) have concluded that an increased risk for unwanted cardiovascular (CV) events has been demonstrated for all the COX-2 selective NSAIDs. The cardiovascular events have a thrombotic nature, being either acute myocardial infarctions (AMI) or strokes. Also, non-selective NSAIDs have a potential of causing unwanted CV events, especially when used in high doses and for longer periods of time.

As a consequence, the Food and Drug Administration (FDA) has requested that all COX-2 selective NSAIDs should be labeled with a boxed warning regarding increased risk of serious CV thrombotic events and a contraindication for patients who have recently undergone a CABG procedure. For non-selective NSAIDs, FDA has concluded that short-term use is not associated with increased CV risk, but the labeling should mention the potential risk [14].

COX-2 selective NSAIDs, especially the coxibs (rofecoxib-removed from market, celecoxib, etoricoxib), inhibit the synthesis of vascular prostacyclin (PGI2), a natural inhibitor of platelet aggregation with vasodilator properties. PGI2 is a protective mediator for cardiovascular system, acting via its receptor IP, expressed in different cell types. The increased risk of vascular events caused by the reduction of PGI2 formation might be mitigated by a simultaneous suppression of COX-1 in the platelets. Unfortunately, COX-2 selective drugs, having no affinity for COX-1, do not reduce the platelet production of thromboxane A2 (TXA2) (**Figure 2**).

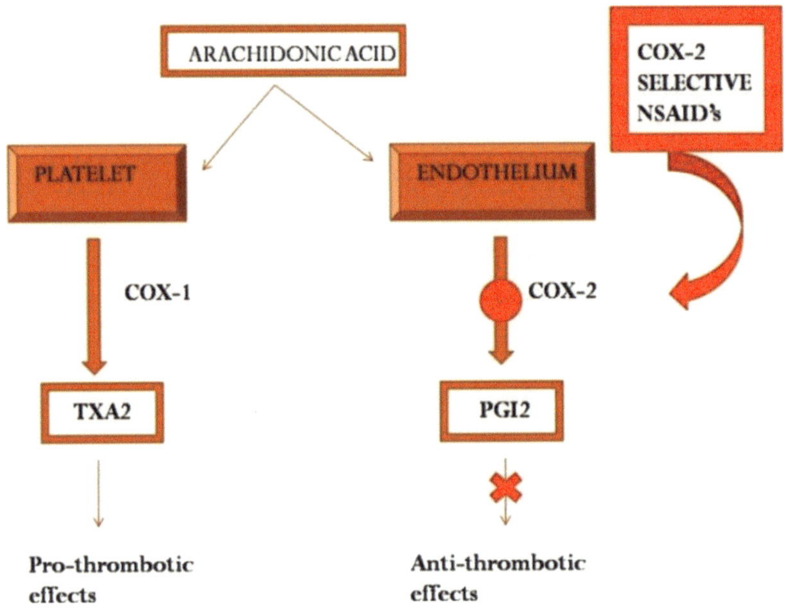

Figure 2. Mechanism of COX-2 selective NSAIDs-induced thrombosis.

Combined, these two effects may lead to a "pro-thrombotic state" with a significant risk of developing myocardial infarction or stroke [5]. However, with the exception of naproxen, neither of the non-selective NSAIDs (apart from aspirin) could affect platelet COX-1 in such a significant manner necessary for a platelet inhibitory effect [15].

Multiple large-scale epidemiological studies have been performed to gather data regarding the cardiovascular (CV) safety profile of the NSAID class.

A comparative analysis of patients with arthritis receiving celecoxib 400 mg twice daily and patients receiving placebo in an aspirin primary prevention meta-analysis showed that the annualized rate for acute myocardial infarction (AMI) was higher in patients receiving celecoxib compared to placebo (0.80 vs. 0.50) [16].

In a meta-analysis of three large observational studies, etoricoxib was associated with a significant 97% increase risk of AMI [17].

For the non-selective drugs, several epidemiological studies have provided conflicting results. For ibuprofen, studies evaluating potential risk for CV events ranged from showing no risk (RR 0.96; 95% CI: 0.81–1.14) to a significantly increased risk (HR 1.84; 95% CI: 1.62–2.08) [18].

For naproxen, studies ranged from showing a decreased risk (RR 0.75; 95% CI: 0.62–0.92) to significantly increased risk (OR 1.27; 95% CI: 1.01–1.60) [19].

More recently, a large meta-analysis of 754 RCTs (350,000 patients) concluded that diclofenac (150 mg daily) presents similar risks to COX-2 selective drugs for mortality (RR 1.02; 95%

CI: 0.84–1.24) but naproxen (1000 mg daily) is associated with fewer CV events and lower mortality [20].

On the basis of evidence gathered so far, several strategies for NSAID treatment and CV prevention have been suggested [5, 14]:

- Patients with low CV risk (under 1%/year) can be administered either a non-selective NSAID or a coxib, the choice between the two depending on the GI risk.
- In patients with intermediate CV risk (1–3%/year), the choice should be ibuprofen or naproxen (+PPI).
- In patients with high CV risk (above 3%/year), the choice is naproxen +PPI and aspirin, given 2 hours before.
- In Europe, EMEA contraindicates coxibs if cardiovascular risk factors are present.

2.3. Renal

In normal human subjects, NSAIDs do not have a significant influence on renal function. Nevertheless, prostaglandins are important mediators at the kidney level. They are involved in maintaining the volume control and electrolyte balance, they also control the release of renin and contribute to renal vasodilation. All NSAIDs can alter renal function by inhibiting COX-1 (which regulates renal hemodynamics and glomerular filtration) and/or COX-2 (which mediates salt and water excretion) expressed in the kidneys [21].

Usually, NSAIDs are associated with salt and water retention, due to the loss of PG-induced action on ADH. This hydro-saline retention has the potential of triggering arterial hypertension, but the effect varies greatly among the different molecules. Apparently, indomethacin and naproxen may increase the mean arterial pressure with 3–4 mm Hg [22].

Rarely, NSAIDs can cause a nephropathy, favored by high doses of multiple drugs but also in patients with congestive heart failure, chronic kidney disease, hypovolemia, disorders of the RAAS system. The manifestations of nephropathy may vary (e.g. interstitial nephritis, nephrotic syndrome, and papillary necrosis), and, unfortunately, it can progress to acute renal failure [23]. Of the available NSAIDs, indomethacin is the most potent inhibitor of renal prostaglandins, therefore being associated with more cases of renal failure. Drugs with an intermediate risk include ibuprofen, naproxen, diclofenac, sulindac, and piroxicam [24]. The nephrotoxic potential of COX-2 selective drugs is less clear.

2.4. Hepatic

Hepatotoxicity is a rare adverse effect of NSAIDs, but with potential serious consequences. A series of clinical trials have reported transient elevations of liver transaminases during the treatment with NSAIDs, but the values have usually normalized in time. Only in a minority of patients, a significant liver injury was observed, with symptoms which included nausea, vomiting, upper abdominal pain, fatigue, and jaundice. The injuries were primarily cholestatic, but hepatocellular or mixed cases were also documented [25].

Two large cohort studies pinpointed a 9/100,000 patients ratio of developing NSAID-associated hepatotoxicity. In the first study, out of 228,392 patients taking diclofenac, indomethacin, naproxen, sulindac, or piroxicam, 34 cases of acute liver injury were identified. The relative risk of developing liver injuries increased in patients with rheumatic diseases (RR 10.9; 95% CI: 2.4–50.2). Age and gender did not increase the relative risk [26]. The second study involved 625,307 patients from England and Wales, only 23 cases of acute liver injury being identified. Only sulindac was associated with a significant risk [27].

Nimesulide, a COX-2 selective NSAID marketed in Europe, was also associated with an increased risk of liver toxicity, but the European Medicines Agency (EMA) concluded in 2011 that the benefit/risk ratio remains positive for patients with acute pain or primary dysmenorrhea [28, 29].

2.5. Blood

Non-steroidal anti-inflammatory drugs (NSAIDs) can affect platelet aggregation and bleeding time due to inhibition of PG and TXA2 synthesis. Aspirin is the most potent compound in this respect, due to the irreversible inhibition of COX-1 from the platelets, which translates into an increase in bleeding time. For aspirin, prolongation of bleeding time is about twice that of baseline in healthy subjects after a single dose of 325 mg. The effect begins 12 hours after a dose, and lasts between 24 and 48 hours. The other drugs from the class can also increase bleeding time, but the values are situated in the upper limit of the normal [30].

2.6. Hypersensitivity

Non-steroidal anti-inflammatory drugs (NSAIDs) have been reported as the second most common cause of drug-induced hypersensitivity reactions, hypersensitivity to aspirin affecting from 0.5 to 1.9% of the general population, with greater prevalence in asthmatics or patients with chronic urticaria [31, 32]. The NSAID-induced hypersensitivity has a wide range of clinical manifestations from anaphylaxis or severe bronchospasm developed within minutes to delayed-type responses, appearing after days or weeks. Bronchial asthma, aspirin-exacerbated respiratory disease (AERD), rhinosinusitis, urticaria are frequently encountered. The delayed-type skin or systemic reactions are very rare and include Stevens-Johnson syndrome, toxic epidermal necrolysis (TEN) and drug reaction with eosinophilia and systemic symptoms (DRESS).

The pathogenetic mechanism of NSAID-induced asthma and AERD is represented by the inhibition of COX-1 (by aspirin and other non-selective NSAIDs), which triggers a mechanism leading to an asthmatic attack or nasal symptoms. Apparently, deprivation of PGE2 may lead to activation of inflammatory pathways and a local and systemic generation of cysteinyl leucotrienes, the most potent bronchoconstrictors.

Beside aspirin, hypersensitivity reactions have been documented especially in NSAIDs with heteroaryl acid group (naproxen, diclofenac, ibuprofen), newer COX-2 selective compounds having a very low incidence of this adverse effect [33].

3. Drug interactions of NSAIDs

Drug interactions are increasingly becoming a major concern for healthcare providers due to the necessity of using multiple drugs for the treatment of complex pathologies [34]. NSAIDs are frequently involved in drug-drug interactions, leading to increased hospitalization and health care cost [35].

3.1. Antihypertensives

In normotensive and untreated hypertensive patients, NSAIDs are probably having a weak effect on blood pressure. The addition of a NSAID to antihypertensive drugs could reduce the efficacy of antihypertensives, with a poor control of blood pressure. Several classes of antihypertensives are more prone to suffer this interaction: renin-angiotensin-aldosterone inhibitors, diuretics, and beta-blockers. Calcium channel blockers and centrally acting sympatholytic drugs are not affected. Elderly patients with hypertension may suffer significant changes in blood pressure control [36].

In addition to effects on blood pressure, there is concern that the interaction NSAID-Antihypertensives could increase the risk of acute kidney injury, since both classes have renal effects [37].

The pathogenetic mechanisms of these interactions are variable. NSAIDs interfere with the angiotensine converting enzyme (ACE) inhibitors directly and indirectly by decreasing renal prostaglandin synthesis and by reducing ACE inhibitors-induced prostaglandin synthesis. Also, NSAIDs decrease the efficacy of diuretics by reducing their natriuretic effect. The beta-blockers are influenced by the reduction of prostaglandin synthesis and a reduction in plasma renin, but their antihypertensive effects are marginally modified [38].

A comprehensive review of clinical data from the USA highlighted that indomethacin, naproxen, and piroxicam were associated with clinically significant increases in blood pressure, especially in patients treated with enalapril [38, 39]. Another US study of hypertensive patients, treated with ACEIs, and also receiving ibuprofen (2400 mg/day), nabumetone (2000 mg/day), or celecoxib (400 mg/day), found that ibuprofen, but not nabumetone or celecoxib, increased the mean arterial pressure with 6.5±1.4 mm Hg [40].

Also, considering that aldosterone antagonists (spironolactone) may increase the risk of GI bleeding, patients should be informed that the long-term use of a NSAID could increase the probability of GI adverse effects [37].

The same US study found that small but significant increases in blood pressure occurred when indomethacin, piroxicam, naproxen, or ibuprofen were introduced in patients treated with hydrochlorothiazide or amiloride [38]. Another study examined the effects of ibuprofen (2400 mg/day) and naproxen (750 mg/day) on blood pressure in hypertensive patients treated with hydrochlorothiazide. After 4 weeks, the effects of NSAIDs on blood pressure were considered minor [41].

In conclusion, hypertensive patients under treatment with ACEIs or hydrochlorothiazide should avoid chronic use of NSAIDs [37].

3.2. Antithrombotics

Drug interactions between NSAIDs and antithrombotic medication have been extensively studied, as they can generate serious consequences.

The simultaneous administration of NSAIDs and cardioprotective aspirin can result in a competition for access into the active site of COX-1. Theoretically, this could lead to a reduction of aspirin's irreversible inhibition of platelet COX-1, with a subsequent reduction of clinical efficacy (prevention of an unwanted thrombotic event). A study on 5208 people found that patients taking prophylactic aspirin together with ibuprofen (more than four times per week) showed an almost doubled risk for MI, compared with patients taking ibuprofen infrequently [42]. Other studies showed different results. A retrospective study on 42,611 patients, including 8688 cases of MI, found that patients treated with aspirin and any NSAID had a lower risk for MI than the ones not taking aspirin and NSAIDs [43]. Another study on 22,071 apparently healthy patients showed that regular but not intermittent use of NSAIDs inhibits the clinical benefits of aspirin [44].

Despite the conflicting results of these studies, the avoidance of chronic use of NSAIDs in patients under treatment with cardioprotective aspirin is advisable. FDA recommends taking ibuprofen at least 8 hours before and 30 minutes after aspirin to reduce the likelihood of an interaction [45].

Although NSAIDs do not cause a direct pharmacodynamic interaction with warfarin, concomitant use may increase the probability of GI bleeding [46].

3.3. Antidepressants

In the 1990s, a large number of reports of bleeding disorders associated with selective serotonin reuptake inhibitors (SSRIs) were published, prompting further investigations. Although platelets do not synthesize serotonin, they can uptake it from plasma, and therefore serotonin may be involved in hemostasis and thrombosis. Thus, at the association of SSRIs with NSAIDs, which can also affect platelets, an interaction is possible. Furthermore, a pharmacokinetic interaction is possible, considering that some SSRIs inhibit CYP2C9, an enzyme involved in the metabolism of ibuprofen and diclofenac [47].

A recent review estimated that the risk of GI bleeding with the use of SSRIs relative to the non-use is 2.6 (95% CI: 1.7–3.8) [48]. Another review of the literature synthesized data from four retrospective studies examining the adverse outcomes from the association of SSRIs with NSAIDs. Two of the studies concluded that the risk ratio for an upper GI bleeding after the association was greater than the additive risk of either drug alone [49].

3.4. Alcohol

Alcohol can favor GI bleeding when consumed in large quantities, so that an additive effect with NSAIDs has been documented. A case-control study using 1224 inpatients found a 2.7- fold increase in the risk for GI bleeding in individuals who regularly took ibuprofen and consumed alcohol (95% CI: 1.6–4.4) [50]. Another study using 1083 hospitalized patients found that the presence of either NSAIDs use or a history of alcohol abuse led to an odds ratio (OR) of 2.9 for severe GI events, while the presence of both risk factors led to an OR of 10.2 [51].

3.5. Methotrexate

Several NSAIDs have been found to reduce renal clearance of methotrexate, which could generate toxic events (renal failure, pancytopenia), especially at high doses [37]. Recently, a Cochrane review stated that using low doses of MTX (under 25 mg weekly, administered sc) and NSAIDs will not produce a clinically significant interaction [52].

4. Conclusions

The non-steroidal anti-inflammatory drugs (NSAIDs) have a variety of clinical applications due to their anti-inflammatory, analgesic, antipyretic, or antithrombotic effects.

The safety profile of NSAIDs remains positive when used in low doses for the temporary relief of pain or fever. In elderly patients, or in those with gastrointestinal or cardiovascular risk factors, more caution is necessary in order to avoid the apparition of serious adverse effects.

Patients chronically treated with ACE inhibitors, hydrochlorothiazide, spironolactone, or aspirin should be informed about the risks of NSAIDs administration.

Author details

Oliviu Vostinaru

Address all correspondence to: oliviu_vostinaru@yahoo.com

Department of Pharmacology, Physiology and Physiopathology, Iuliu Hatieganu University of Medicine and Pharmacy, Cluj-Napoca, Romania

References

[1] Grosser T, Smyth E, FitzGerald GA. Anti-inflammatory, antipyretic and analgesic agents; Pharmacotherapy of Gout. In: Brunton LL, Chabner BA, Knollmann BC editors. Goodman and Gillman's The Pharmacological Basis of Therapeutics, 12th ed. McGraw Hill Medical; 2011. pp. 959-976.

[2] Vane JR. Inhibition of prostaglandin synthesis as a mechanism of action for Aspirin-like drugs. Nat New Biol. 1971; 231:232-235.

[3] FitzGerald GA, Patrono C. The coxibs, selective inhibitors of cyclooxygenase-2. NEJM. 2001; 345:433-442.

[4] Pirmohamed M, James S, Meakin S, Green C, Scott AK, Walley TJ. Adverse drug reaction as cause of admission to hospital: prospective analysis of 18820 patients. BMJ. 2004; 329:15-19.

[5] Patrignani P, Tacconelli S, Bruno A, Sostres C, Lanas A. Managing the adverse effects of non-steroidal anti-inflammatory drugs. Expert Rev Clin Pharmacol. 2011; 4(5):605-621.

[6] Lazzaroni M, Bianchi Porro G. Gastrointestinal side-effects of traditional non-steroidal anti-inflammatory drugs and new formulations. Aliment Pharmacol Ther. 2004; 20(2):48-58.

[7] Singh G, Triadafilopoulos G. Epidemiology of NSAID-induced GI complications. J Rheumatol. 1999; 26:18-24.

[8] Gabriel SE, Jaakkimainen L. Bombardier C. Risk of serious gastrointestinal complications related to use of NSAID's: a meta-analysis. Ann Intern Med. 1991; 115:787-796.

[9] Russel RI. Defining patients at risk of non-steroidal anti-inflammatory gastropathy. Ital J Gastroenterol Hepatol. 1999; 31(1):14-18.

[10] Moore N, Vanganse E, Leparc JM et al. The PAIN study: Paracetamol, aspirin and ibuprofen new tolerability study: a large scale randomised clinical trial comparing the tolerability of aspirin, ibuprofen and paracetamol for short term analgesia. Clin Drug Investig. 1999; 18(2):89-98.

[11] Silverstein FE, Faich G, Goldstein JL et al. Gastrointestinal toxicity with celecoxib vs. non-steroidal anti-inflammatory drugs for osteoarthritis and rheumatoid arthritis. The CLASS study: a randomised control trial. JAMA. 2000; 284:1247-1255.

[12] Curtis SP, Lee M, Ng J et al. Fewer upper-GI perforations, ulcers and bleeds (PUBs) with etoricoxib than with non-selective cyclooxygenase inhibitors (NSAID's). Ann Rheum Dis. 2002; 61:177.

[13] Hooper L, Brown TJ, Elliot R et al. The effectiveness of five strategies for the prevention of gastrointestinal toxicity induced by non-steroidal anti-inflammatory drugs: systematic review BMJ. 2004; 329:948-957.

[14] Summary Minutes of the Joint Arthritis Advisory Committee and Drug Safety and Risk Management Advisory Committee Meeting February 10-11, 2014. Silver Spring, MD: Food and Drug Administration; Center for Drug Evaluation and Research; 2014. Available from: http://www.fda.gov/downloads/AdvisoryCommittees/CommitteesMeetingMaterials/Drugs/ArthritisAdvisoryCommittee/UCM395527.pdf.

[15] Capone ML, Tacconelli S, Sciulli MG et al. Human pharmacology of naproxen sodium. J Pharmacol Exp Ther. 2007; 322:453-460.

[16] Mukherjee D, Nissen SE, Topol EJ. Risk of cardiovascular events associated with selective COX-2 inhibitors. JAMA. 2001; 286(8):954-959.

[17] Varas-Lorenzo C, Riera-Guardia N, Calingaert B et al. Myocardial infarction and individual non-steroidal anti-inflammatory drugs meta-analysis of observational studies. Pharmacoepidemiol Drug Saf. 2013; 22(6):559-570.

[18] Fosbøl EL, Gislason GH, Jacobsen S et al. Risk of myocardial infarction and death associated with the use of nonsteroidal anti-inflammatory drugs (NSAIDs) among healthy individuals: a nationwide cohort study. Clin Pharmacol Ther. 2009; 85(2): 190-197.

[19] Hippisley-Cox J, Coupland C. Risk of myocardial infarction in patients taking cyclo-oxygenase-2 inhibitors or conventional non-steroidal anti-inflammatory drugs: population based nested case-control analysis. BMJ. 2005; 330(7504):1366.

[20] Coxib and traditional NSAID's Trialists Colaboration. Vascular and upper gastrointestinal effects of non-steroidal anti-inflammatory drugs: meta-analysis of individual participant data from randomized trials. Lancet. 2013; 382:769-779.

[21] Weir MR. Renal effects of nonselective NSAIDs and coxibs. Cleve Clin J Med. 2002; 69(Suppl 1):SI53-SI58.

[22] Pope JE, Anderson JJ, Felson DT. A meta-analysis of the effects of nonsteroidal anti-inflammatory drugs on blood pressure. Arch Intern Med. 1993; 153(4):477-484.

[23] Whelton A. Renal and related cardiovascular effects of conventional and COX-2 specific NSAID's and non-NSAID analgesics. Am J Therap. 2000; 7:63-74.

[24] Piepho R, Whelton A, Mayor G et al. Clinical therapeutic conference. J Clin Pharmacol. 1991; 31:785-791.

[25] Prescott LF. Effect of non-narcotic analgesics on the liver. Drugs. 1986; 32(4):129-147.

[26] Garcia Rodriguez LA, Williams R, Derby LE et al. Acute liver injury associated with non-steroidal anti-inflammatory drugs and the role of risk factors. Arch Intern Med. 1994; 154:311-316

[27] Garcia Rodriguez LA, Gutthann SP, Walker AM et al. The role of non-steroidal anti-inflammatory drugs in acute liver injury. BMJ. 1992; 305:865-868.

[28] Cazacu I, Mogosan C, Loghin F. Safety issues of current analgesics: an update. Clujul Medical. 2015; 88(2):128-136.

[29] European Medicines Agency. EMA concludes review of systemic nimesulide-containing medicines. Use to be restricted to treatment of acute pain and primary dysmenorrhoea. 2011. Available from: http://www.ema.europa.eu/docs/en_GB/document_library/Press_release/2011/06/WC500107903.pdf.

[30] Schafer AI. Effects of nonsteroidal anti-inflammatory drugs on platelet function and systemic hemostasis. J Clin Pharmacol. 1995; 35:209-219.

[31] Gomes ER, Demoly P. Epidemiology of hypersensitivity drug reactions. Curr Opin Allergy Clin Immunol. 2005; 5:309-316.

[32] Settipane RA, Constantine HP, Settipane GA. Aspirin intolerance and recurrent urticaria in normal adults and children. Epidemiology and review. Allergy. 1980; 35:149-154.

[33] Kowalski ML, Makowska JS, Blanca M et al. Hypersensitivity to nonsteroidal anti-inflammatory drugs (NSAID's)-classification, diagnosis and management: review of the EAACI/ENDA and GA2LEN/HANNA. Allergy. 2011; 66:818-829.

[34] Bucsa CD, Cazacu I, Farcas AM, Bojita M. The prevalence of potential drug-drug interactions in the therapy of Romanian community pharmacy's patients. Farmacia. 2012; 60(4):510-516.

[35] Shad MU, Marsh C, Preskorn SH. The economic consequences of a drug-drug interaction. J Clin Psychopharmacol. 2001; 21:119-120.

[36] Mene P, Pugliese F, Patrono C. The effects of non-steroidal anti-inflammatory drugs on human hypertensive vascular disease. Sem Nephrol. 1995; 15:244-252.

[37] Moore N, Pollack C, Butkerait P. Adverse drug reactions and drug-drug interactions with over-the-counter NSAID's. Ther Clin Risk Manag. 2015; 11:1061-1075.

[38] McFarlane LL, Orak DJ, Simpson WM. NSAID's, antihypertensive agents and loss of blood pressure control. Am Fam Physician. 1995; 51:849-856.

[39] Armstrong EP, Malone DC. The impact of nonsteroidal anti-inflammatory drugs on blood pressure with an emphasis on newer agents. Clin Therap. 2003; 25(1):1-18.

[40] Palmer R, Weiss R, Zusman RM, Haig A, Flavin S, McDonald B. Effects of nabumetone, celecoxib and ibuprofen on blood pressure control in hypertensive patients on angiotensine converting enzyme inhibitors. Am J Hypertens. 2003; 16(2):135-139.

[41] Klassen D, Goodfriend TL, Schuna AA, Young DY, Peterson CA. Assessment of blood pressure during treatment with naproxen or ibuprofen in hypertensive patients treated with hydrochlorothiazide. J Clin Pharmacol. 1993; 33(10):971-978.

[42] Kimmel SE, Berlin JA, Reilly M et al. The effects on nonselective non-aspirin non-steroidal anti-inflammatory medications on the risk of nonfatal myocardial infarction and their interaction with aspirin. J Am Coll Cardiol. 2004; 43(6):985-990.

[43] Fischer LM, Schlienger RG, Matter CM, Jick H, Meier CR. Current use of nonsteroidal anti-inflammatory drugs and the risk of myocardial infarction. Pharmacotherapy. 2005; 25(4):503-510.

[44] Kurth T, Glynn RJ, Walker AM, Chan KA, Buring JE, Hennekens CH, Gaziano JM. Inhibition of clinical benefits of aspirin on first myocardial infarction by nonsteroidal anti-inflammatory drugs. Circulation. 2003; 108(10):1191-1195.

[45] Food and Drug Administration. Information for Healthcare Professionals: Concomitant use of ibuprofen and aspirin. Silver Spring, MD: U.S. Food and Drug Administration; 2006 [updated August 14, 2013]. Available from: http://www.fda.gov/Drugs/DrugSafety/Postmarket Drug Safety Information for Patients and Providers/ucm125222.htm.

[46] Mellemkjaer L, Blot WJ, Sørensen HT et al. Upper gastrointestinal bleeding among users of NSAIDs: a population-based cohort study in Denmark. Br J Clin Pharmacol. 2002; 53(2):173-181.

[47] Zullino DF, Khazaal Y. Increased risk of gastrointestinal adverse effects under SSRI/NSAID combination may be due to pharmacokinetic interactions. Br J Clin Pharmacol. 2005; 59(1):118-119.

[48] DeAbajo FJ, Montero D, Rodriguez LA et al. Antidepressants and risk of upper gastrointestinal bleeding. Basic Clin Pharmacol Toxicol 2006; 98(3):304-310.

[49] Mort JR, Aparasu RR, Baer RK. Interaction between selective serotonin reuptake inhibitors and nonsteroidal antiinflammatory drugs: review of the literature. Pharmacotherapy. 2006; 26(9):1307-1313.

[50] Kaufman DW, Kelly JP, Wiholm BE et al. The risk of acute major upper gastrointestinal bleeding among users of aspirin and ibuprofen at various levels of alcohol consumption. Am J Gastroenterol. 1999; 94(11):3189-3196.

[51] Neutel CI, Appel WC. The effects of alcohol abuse on the risk of NSAID-related gastrointestinal events. Ann Epidemiol. 2000; 10(4):246-250.

[52] Colebatch AN, Marks JL, van der Heijde DM, Edwards CJ. Safety of nonsteroidal antiinflammatory drugs and/or paracetamol in people receiving methotrexate for inflammatory arthritis: a Cochrane systematic review. J Rheumatol. 2012; 90:62-73.

Chapter 4

NSAID$_S$: Design and Development of Innovative Oral Delivery Systems

Giulia Auriemma, Andrea Cerciello and
Rita P. Aquino

Additional information is available at the end of the chapter

http://dx.doi.org/10.5772/intechopen.68240

Abstract

Recently, different technologies have been used to transform active pharmaceutical ingredients (APIs) into new dosage forms. Engineered drug delivery systems may modify biopharmaceutical properties of the API achieving either immediate or delayed release according to specific therapeutic needs. Particularly, preprogrammed release of oral formulations delivering the drug at expected times may be useful in chronotherapy of early morning pathologies. The conventional approach when dealing with such diseases is to administer NSAIDs two to three times daily. This approach does not allow to fit drug release with symptoms onset resulting in inefficient therapy and poor patient compliance. NSAIDs may be very effective if administered at least 4–6 h before the pain reaches its peak in the early morning. The solution could be to design delayed drug delivery systems allowing one administration before going to sleep acting in the early morning. This chapter highlights new approaches in developing controlled delivery systems of NSAIDs potentially useful to treat both acute and chronic inflammation. The chapter illustrates the versatility of laminar jet break-up technology (prilling) to produce gel beads able to control rate and time of drug delivery. A special focus will be on particle-engineering strategies, i.e., prilling and prilling technique in tandem with microwave or supercritical fluid-assisted drying.

Keywords: oral drug delivery, modified release dosage forms, chronotherapy, early morning pathologies, NSAIDs, prilling; hydrogels drying, dissolution, *in vivo* effectiveness

1. Introduction

Any drug delivery system (DDS) may be defined as a system comprising:

- active pharmaceutical ingredients (APIs) and
- medical device or dosage form able to carry the drug inside the body.

To obtain a therapeutic response, the suitable amount of the drug must be delivered at the right time, in a safe and reproducible manner, to a specific target and at the required level. The distribution of the drug to tissues different from the sites of action and organs of elimination is a potential cause of toxicity.

Innovative drug delivery systems may overcome problems commonly related to conventional formulations. In fact, in the last few years, there is a continuous research in the development of engineered particles and systems for the targeted delivery and/or controlled release of APIs. These systems can protect the drug from degradation, realize controlled release, modify pharmacokinetics and biodistribution profiles, reduce clearance and side effects, and improve drug specificity. The administration of an old drug through an engineered delivery system may contribute to the improvement of the drug efficacy, safety, and patient compliance and may extend its conventional clinical applications [1, 2]. For example, in the treatment of both acute (i.e., postoperative pain, dental surgery) and chronic inflammatory diseases, immediate or delayed drug delivery systems are essential.

The development of delivery systems able to control and delay drug release is acquiring a growing interest with the recent advances in chronopharmacology. In fact, treating diseases affected by the circadian rhythms, such as "early morning pathologies" (EMPs) (rhinitis, rheumatoid arthritis, etc.) [3–5], requires a desired concentration of drug available at expected times [6, 7]. This effect may be assured by device releasing no drug within the time gap and delivering the optimal amount at certain point correspondent to symptoms peak [8–10]. Diseases with established circadian cycle show day–night patterns in the onset and symptoms exacerbation, usually with peaks in the morning and decrease throughout day [11]. Moreover, the plasma concentration of C-reactive protein and interleukin-6 has been shown to follow a circadian rhythm in chronic inflammatory-based diseases such as rheumatoid arthritis [12]. The main goals when dealing with such pathologies are as follows: stop inflammation, relieve symptoms, improve physical function and overall well-being, and reduce long-term complications.

Nonsteroidal anti-inflammatory drugs (NSAIDs) represent one of the most used classes of drugs in the management of EMPs. These molecules inhibit COX and prevent further formation of prostaglandins and other related inflammatory mediators. Based on their mechanism of action, NSAIDs are useful as adjuvant therapy for the symptomatic management of the diseases, reducing inflammation and pain. NSAIDs employed to relieve symptoms are usually administered to patients through oral route at different moment of the day (after awakening, after lunch, and during the night) through immediate-release formulations. In this way, drugs are rapidly absorbed and explicate their action independently from the circadian rhythms of hormones and cytokines responsible of EMP symptomatology. Such a conventional approach usually leads to ineffective therapy because drug liberation from the dosage form is not synchronized with the symptom peak resulting in an increase in side effects and, consequently, poor patient compliance. This explains why in the last few years a growing number of researchers have focused on the possibility to treat EMPs with a chronotherapeutic approach through oral route.

NSAIDs (i.e., indomethacin, aceclofenac, ketoprofen, flurbiporfen, and lornoxicam) are attractive API to be modified in their formulation obtaining chronotherapeutic drug delivery systems (ChDDSs) useful in the treatment of early morning pathologies [13]. For example, a pH-responsive dual pulse multiparticulate dosage form containing ketoprofen was developed and tested in rheumatoid arthritis. Results showed that this formulation was able to relieve circadian symptoms during midnight and early morning [14]. Levi et al. observed that the evening administration of indomethacin in a controlled release formulation was able to better control morning symptoms compared to the same formulation administered in other moment of the day [15].

Among different approaches used to design pharmaceutical dosage forms tailored to follow the human chronobiological rhythm [10, 16, 17], micro-technologies have been applied as innovative and efficient tool [18, 19]. Several methods and techniques are potentially useful for the preparation of polymeric microparticles, such as spray drying, fluid bed coating, solvent evaporation, coacervation phase separation, prilling, etc. The choice of a specific microencapsulation technology is related to the polymer nature, the chemical features of drug, the desired particles size, as well as to the reproducibility and ease to scale ability of the method [20].

1.1. Prilling technique

Among the different processes used for the preparation of ChDDSs, prilling or laminar jet breakup technique is an emerging process able to produce homogenous microparticles with high drug content and controlled release properties. Prilling is a vibration-based technology consisting in breaking apart a laminar jet of polymer solution into a row of monosized drops by means of a vibrating nozzle device (**Figure 1**) [21, 22]. Once the droplets are formed, the gelation/consolidation step follows in order to prevent either the aggregation of polymer droplets or the undesired leakage of encapsulated drugs. The chemical nature of the droplets (dispersed phase) determines the consolidation step, in which the droplets are transformed into solid microparticles known as gel-beads; this procedure can involve temperature modification, chemical reactions, and mainly ionic cross-linking (ionotropic gelation).

Several variables in prilling can affect droplet size and size distribution as polymer concentration and flow rate [23, 24], frequency of vibration, as well as falling distance. In fact, using high wavelengths of the jet breakup and reducing the falling distance to the hardening solution, the drop coalescence can be reduced. Thus, smaller nozzle diameters and higher frequencies increase the possibility of coalescence [22]. The frequency is usually kept as low as possible in order to avoid the formation of satellite droplets leading to a broader size range [21]. The

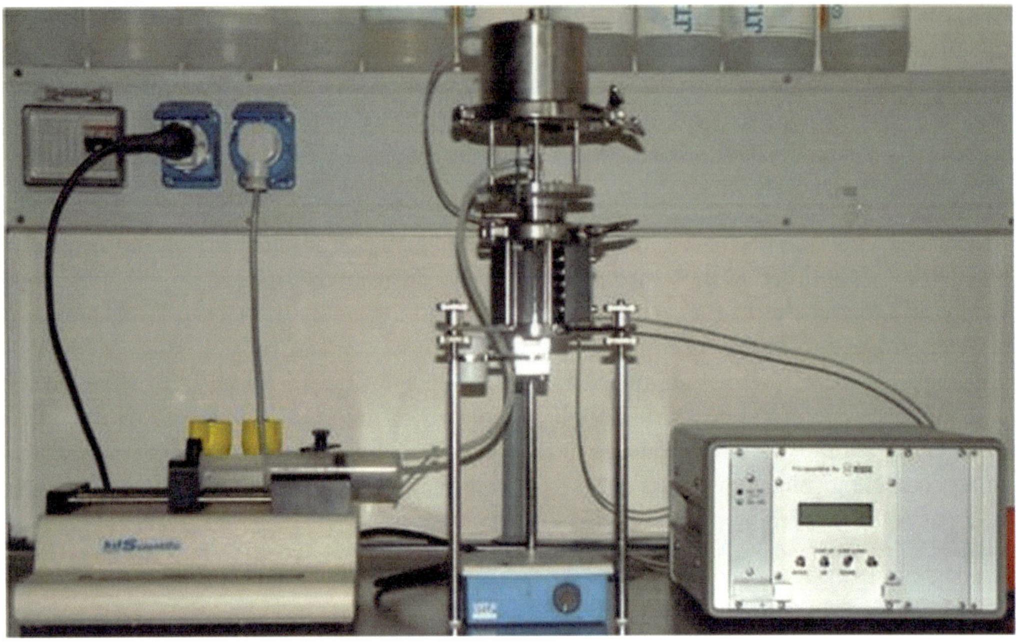

Figure 1. Prilling apparatus (Nisco Inc.) at the Department of Pharmacy, University of Salerno.

production of microparticles by the vibrating nozzle device is highly reproducible, is time-saving, and can be performed under aseptic and scaled-up conditions [25]. The acoustic jet excitation process involved in prilling was patented for production of uniform microspheres of alginate [26], collagen [27], and PLGA [28, 29]. The scale-up of the vibration process may be done by using a multinozzle system (**Figure 2**) without changing other process parameters such as flow rate and the vibration frequency [30]. However, the arrangement of the nozzles which must ensure equal jet formation and equal pressure drops between the nozzles is an

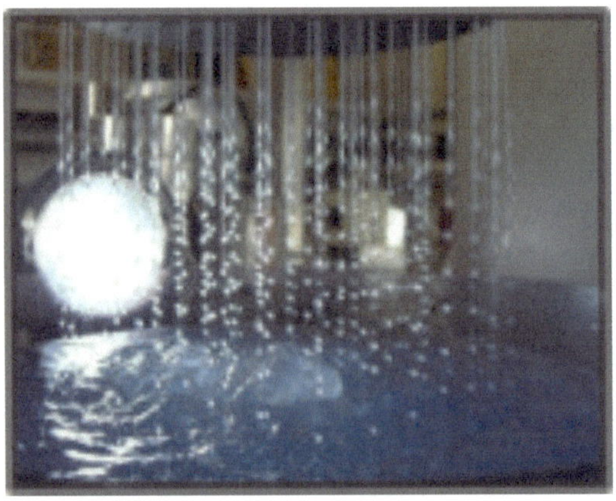

Figure 2. Multinozzle system BRACE GmbH [32].

important parameter [30]. The pilot apparatus using this technique is now being sold by Brace GmbH (Germany), Nisco Inc. (Switzerland), and Inotech AG (Switzerland) [22, 31].

The ionotropic gelation, a highly used consolidation step, is based on the ability of polyelectrolyte polymers (alginate, pectin, chitosan, and gellan gum) to cross-link in the presence of counter ions [32, 33]. Divalent cations (Cd^{2+}, Co^{2+}, Cu^{2+}, Mn^{2+}, Ni^{2+}, Pb^{2+}, and Zn^{2+}) are suitable cross-linking agents with the exception of Mg^{2+} [32, 33]. The binding affinity depends on the chemical composition of the selected polysaccharide, which varies with the source, the characteristics of the polyvalent cations (i.e., ionic radius and coordination number), and the presence of water of hydration surrounding cross-linking ions [32].

After the production stage, hydrogels require to be dried to avoid chemical or microbiological degradation [34]. Drying processes may have a different impact on the final properties of the dried product (solute migration, polymorphism, damages by overheating, and structural modifications). Therefore, the selection of drying technique has a crucial role to determine the textural of the final product and to avoid altering its quality.

2. Prilling-based tandem techniques to produce NSAIDs controlled delivery systems

In this chapter, we described three different prilling-based tandem techniques to produce chronotherapeutic dosage forms delivering NSAIDs. The techniques are based on the combination of prilling with conventional drying, microwave-assisted drying, or supercritical fluid-assisted drying [35].

2.1. Prilling in tandem with conventional drying

To effectively formulate NSAIDs targeting EMPs, prilling microtechnology in combination with conventional drying was used. The traditional drying of hydrogels is based on the evaporation of the solvent; when the solvent inside the pores of the material evaporates, they are subjected to high tension, which causes the partial collapsing of the structure and the wet gel is changed in the so-called "xerogel." Usually, this process is rapid, cheap, and easy to perform. Furthermore, recent studies [36–39] suggested that the opportune setup of some drying parameters may allow the production of materials with unique structural properties, i.e., microporous, micro-mesoporous, or micro-macroporous systems.

In this section, we described the combination of prilling technique with conventional drying to obtain xerogel-based beads loaded with ketoprofen, ketoprofen lysine salt, and piroxicam.

2.1.1. Ketoprofen-loaded xerogels as new ChDDSs: design and in vitro/in vivo characterization

Ketoprofen is a NSAID commonly used in some EMPs as rheumatoid arthritis for its analgesic and anti-inflammatory features. Nevertheless, many collateral effects, such as gastric troubles, restrict its therapeutic benefit. Furthermore, its short biological half-life ($t_{1/2}$= 2.1h) and the need of a high number of daily administrations enhance side effects especially for chronic therapy. For these reasons, ketoprofen is a good candidate for the development of controlled release formulations, able to provide drug release at predetermined rate and time, targeting intestine [21, 40].

2.1.1.1. Approach #1

With the aim to delay ketoprofen release as needed for chronotherapy of EMPs, we designed a gel-beads formulation for delayed delivery of ketoprofen release and *in vivo* absorption for several hours [41, 42].

2.1.1.1.1. Methods

The engineered particles were produced by prilling/ionotropic gelation technique using alginate as gastroresistant polymer carrier and zinc as cross-linking agent. Particularly, Zn^{2+} was also selected for its anti-oxidant properties that may boost the efficacy of the anti-inflammatory drug encapsulated in the polymeric matrix [43, 44]. After the production, hydrated particles were then exposed to standard room conditions (22 °C; 67% RH) for 12–18 h until constant weight was reached obtaining xerogel beads. During the work, different experiments were conducted for the optimization of process parameters in order to obtain ketoprofen gel-beads with desired properties and performances (**Table 1**). Beads micromeritics, solid state, and drug release properties were studied using established method (SEM, DSC, USP 36 Paddle Dissolution).

2.1.1.1.2. Results and discussion

Formulation AK_5 obtained with the highest ketoprofen content (alginate 2% w/w; ketoprofen–alginate ratio = 1:5) showed the highest value of both actual drug content (ADC 9%) and encapsulation efficiency (EE 53%). It is interesting to point out that ADC and EE were related to the drug/polymer ratios suggesting that the incorporation of a great quantity of ketoprofen (into the feed solutions) could induce, during the gelation process, the establishment of intermolecular interactions (as hydrophobic or hydrogen bonding) able to stabilize the "egg-box" structure, leading to a more strong cross-linked matrix. All K-loaded beads exhibited a remarkable reduction in mean diameter in comparison to blank beads with diameters' values

Alginate concentration = 2.0% (w/w)	**Gelling cations = Zn^{2+}**
Drug/polymer ratio = 1:20–1:10–1:5	Gelling time = 2 min
Ø nozzle = 400 μm	pH gelling solution =1.5
N = 0.350 kHz A = 100%	Flow rate = 5 mL/min

Composition of the aqueous feed solutions, prilling parameters (nozzle diameter Ø, frequency N and amplitude A of vibration, and flow rate), gelling solution variables (divalent cation for ionotropic gelling, pH of the gelling solution and cross-linking time).

Table 1. Optimized prilling operative conditions.

http://dx.doi.org/10.5772/intechopen.68240

in the range of 1.7–1.8 mm. Stabilization of the polymer matrix influenced beads shape after the drying process. In particular, SEM analyses confirmed that K-loaded beads had almost spherical shape according to K loading (**Figure 3**).

Pilot dissolution tests of all formulations were performed by conventional vessel methods (USP Apparatus 2, paddle) [45] using a classic pH change method, providing essential information and recommended in various guidelines [46] as a first choice for the *in vitro* dissolution testing of controlled/modified release formulations [47]. Results showed that AK_5 exhibited a gastroresistant profile followed by a slow and extended release of K in SIF (**Figure 4A**). Probably, the intermolecular interactions combined to the high zinc ability to cross-link alginate moieties, led to a strong polymeric matrix for AK_5 able to better control the drug diffusion. The dissolution profile of this formulation was deeply studied using the USP apparatus 4 (flow-through, open-loop configuration), because, as reported in literature, it is able to accurately mimic *in vivo* hydrodynamics and consequently better predict the real *in vivo* behavior of oral formulations [48, 49]. USP apparatus 4 analysis (**Figure 4B**), confirmed the enteric release ability of AK_5 beads showing in SIF a slower ketoprofen release compared to USP 2 analysis. The observed differences were mainly due to the particular hydrodynamic conditions realized by the USP 4 apparatus (no agitation mechanism and constant exposure to the formulation to a laminar flow) that are very similar to the *in vivo* gastrointestinal conditions [50, 51].

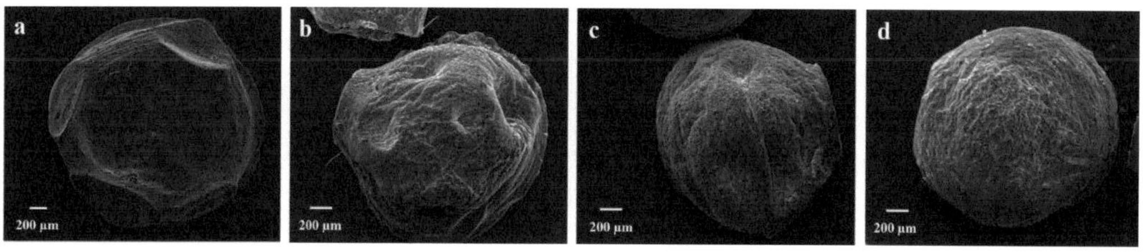

Figure 3. SEM microphotographs of dried Zn-alginate beads formulations: (a) blank beads, (b) AK_20, (c) AK_10, and (d) AK_5.

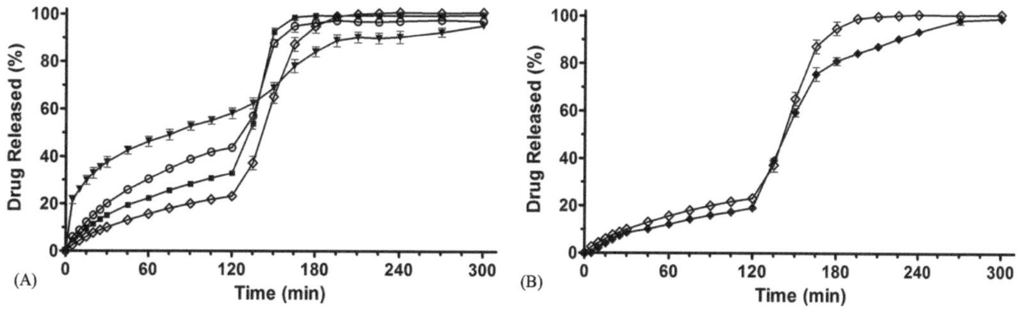

Figure 4. (A) Release profiles of K raw material (-▾-) and K-loaded formulations AK_20 (-o-), AK_10 (-▪-), and AK_5 (-◇-), performed by USP Apparatus 2; (B) release profiles comparison of AK_5 obtained by USP Apparatus 2 (-◇-) and USP Apparatus 4 (-◆-), using a pH change assay. Mean ± SD; (n=6).

To verify whether the *in vitro* drug release may be correlated to a prolonged anti-inflammatory effectiveness, AK_5 (ketoprofen equivalent dose of 3 mg/kg) was tested *in vivo* using a carrageenan-induced acute edema in rat paw (male Wistar rats). Its activity was compared to the activity of pure drug. In detail, samples were administered to rats at the time 5, 3, and 0.5 h before the injection of the phlogistic agent, and paw volume was measured plethysmographycally at the time zero, each hour for 6 h, and at 24 h.

As shown in **Figure 5**, AK_5 exhibited a prolonged anti-inflammatory effect expressed as paw volume reduction, after oral administration in rats in comparison with the control. Unformulated ketoprofen (3 mg/kg) reduced rat paw edema only with a contemporary administration (0.5 h before carrageenan injection), without any effect at t=3 or 5 h before the phlogistic agent injection. Blank zinc-alginate beads, administered to rats at the same time points, did not interfere with the inflammatory process. AK_5 administered 3 or 5 h before edema induction still showed a significant anti-inflammatory activity reducing maximum paw volume (3–4 h) in response to carrageenan injection, therefore reflecting its drug delayed release (**Figures 4** and **5**). Moreover, the prolonged *in vivo* anti-inflammatory effect may be related to the mucoadhesive features of alginate particles able to reduce the ketoprofen absorption in the gastrointestinal tract [52].

Being the optimized formulation AK_5 able to delay *in vivo* K release and absorption up to 6–7 h, it can be considered a potential chronotherapeutic system for the delivery of K. Opportunely timing its administration is possible to match the disease rhythms and to control early morning symptoms in inflammatory-based EMPs.

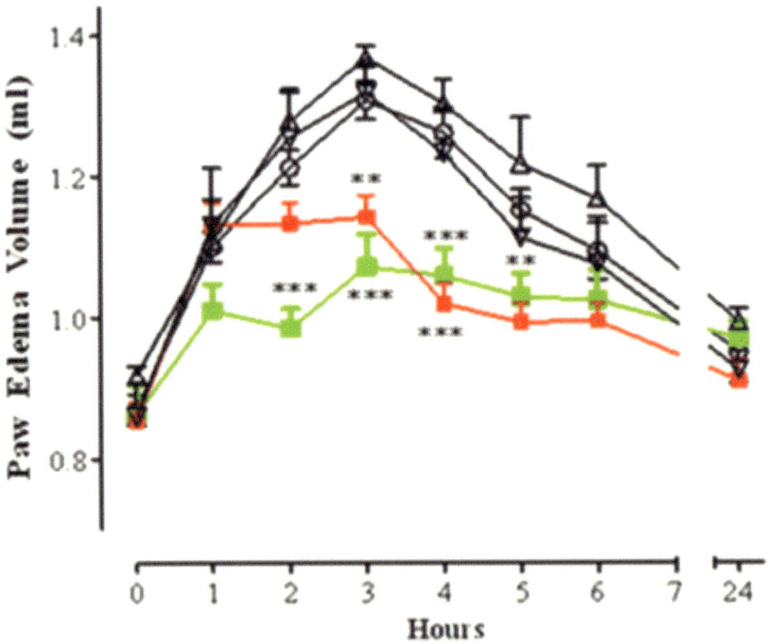

Figure 5. Edema volume reduction obtained administering AK_5 and pure K per *os* to rats 5h (-■-_AK_5 and -∇-_K) and 3h (-■-_AK_5 and -Δ-_K) before carrageenan injection compared to control (-o-); mean ± SD (n=8). **P ≤ 0.01, ***P ≤ 0.001 compared with control.

http://dx.doi.org/10.5772/intechopen.68240

2.1.1.2. Approach #2

These preliminary results have been the starting point to further improve technological properties of gel-beads' formulations in terms of ketoprofen loading and release performances. Therefore, in the following study, we designed a more complex system based on core/shell particles (double-layered particles) consisting of a Zn-pectinate core loading NSAID and an enteric shell of Eudragit S100 (anionic copolymer of methacrylic acid and methyl methacrylate insoluble in acid pH) [53]. Among different commercially available pectins, we focused our attention on amidated low methoxy (ALM) pectin (esterification degree 24% and amidation degree 23%) that, showing high hydrophobic interactions between pectin chains and internal hydrogen bonding between amide groups, is able to stabilize the egg-box structure [54]. Pectins are usually classified on the basis of their degree of esterification (DE) and divided in high methoxyl (HM_DE > 50%) and low methoxyl pectin (LM_ DE< 50%). The latter are the most suitable for the development of oral controlled drug delivery systems. In addition, as reported in the literature, the presence of amide groups in low methoxyl pectin enhances the gel-forming ability, the stability under different pH conditions improving, consequently, the possibility to control drug release [55].

2.1.1.2.1. Methods

Ketoprofen-loaded core particles based on Zn-pectinate matrix were produced by prilling technique using optimized operative conditions [53]. Beads micromeritics, solid state, and drug release properties were studied using established method (SEM, DSC, USP 36 Paddle Dissolution).

2.1.1.2.2. Results and discussion

Formulation BK_5 (Pectin 6% w/w, drug/polymer ratio = 1:5), obtained with the greatest amount of drug, showed the best morphology and the highest EE value (86.7%). In fact, as also observed for alginate beads loaded with ketoprofen [41], the drug and its amount play an important role during the gel matrix formation conditioning and therefore affect technological and mechanic properties of the final dosage form.

To obtain information about *in vitro* release performances, this formulation was tested through a USP apparatus II using a classic pH change method. As expected, monolayered Zn-pectinate beads were not properly effective in retaining drug in simulated gastric fluid (22.2% of the drug was released in 120 min). Their solubility and swelling properties in aqueous media allow a prompt release of NSAID after the pH change of the dissolution fluid (complete drug release was achieved in 180 min). The chronotherapeutic system was obtained by coating zinc-pectinate core (BK_5) with a Eudragit S100® shell. The core–shell system BK_5/E40, obtained applying coating in the amount of 40% (w/w), showed a strong delay of ketoprofen release in SGF followed by a slow and controlled release in SIF (**Figure 6**). This system was able to significantly reduce ketoprofen release in acidic environment from 22.2% (BK_5) up to 7.3% and to prolong its release in simulated intestinal medium. In fact, after the pH change, drug release was completed in approximately 3 h (t=300 min) rather than in 1 h (t= 180) as for BK_5. Only after the dissolution of the enteric shell in SIF, the zinc-pectinate core is exposed to the fluid and pectin chains begin the hydrolysis, releasing slowly the loaded drug. This profile appears feasible and potentially effective for chronotherapy of early morning pathologies.

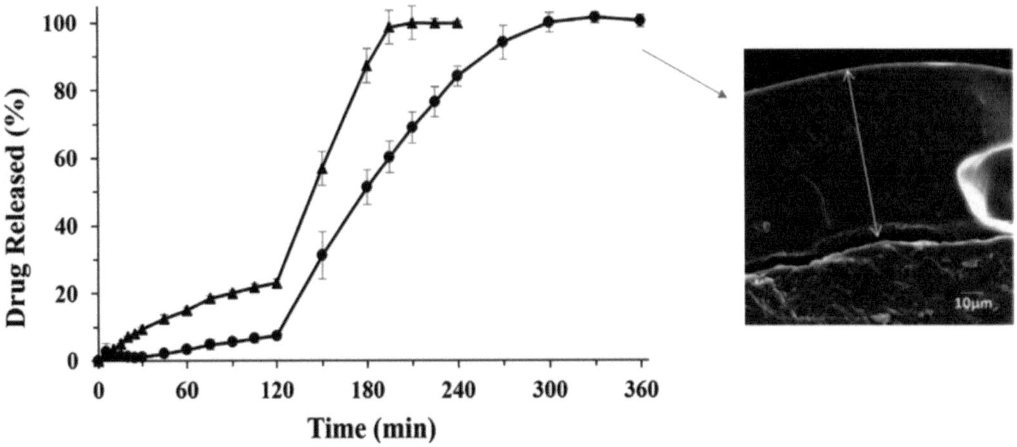

Figure 6. Drug release profiles of core–shell system BK5/E40 (-●-) compared to monolayer formulation BK5 (-▲-) and SEM picture of a cryo-fractured core–shell particle BK5/E40 with magnification of the core–shell structure.

2.1.2. Ketoprofen lysine salt-loaded beads: design and characterization

Although several studies have been reported on polysaccharide hydrogels entrapping the nonsoluble form of ketoprofen [21, 41, 53, 56], few data are available on its L-lysine salt showing better pharmacokinetics and tolerability, enhancement in the rate of absorption, reduction of the onset of therapeutic effect, as well as improvement of the gastric tolerance [57]. The major issue encountered when dealing with such API is the high aqueous solubility preventing the formulation of delivery systems with high encapsulation efficiency values and, above all, effective controlled release properties [58].

Thanks to the expertise grew up in the last few years, we proposed alginate and ALM pectin as carriers and release tailoring agents for the development by prilling of chronotherapeutic system loaded with KL. As highly soluble drugs in hydrogels exhibit poor drug entrapment and ineffective control in drug release, many formulation variables have been investigated to find the optimal ones.

2.1.2.1. Methods

Beads were prepared using Zn^{2+} as a gelling agent and optimizing cross-linking conditions as follows: temperature (4–5°C), pH (1.5) and gelling time (2 min). Different formulations were produced setting polymer concentration at 2.0% and 6.0% w/w for alginate (A) or pectin (B), respectively, and varying drug-polymer ratio as follows: 1:20 (KL_20), 1:10 (KL_10) and 1:5 (KL_5). Drying process of the hydrated beads was conducted by exposing them to standard room conditions as previously described. Beads micromeritics, solid state, and drug release properties were studied using established method (SEM, DSC, USP 36 Paddle Dissolution).

2.1.2.2. Results and discussion

ADC and EE values were related to the specific polymeric material used (A or B) and drug polymer ratio. The higher the drug polymer ratio, the higher the EE. KL encapsulation was higher in pectin (81–94%) than in alginate (39–49%) beads. This effect could be related to the low molecular weight of pectin able to improve the hydrogel structure [59, 60]. The produced particles were cryofractured and analyzed by SEM (**Figure 7**) with the aim to study the effect of alginate or pectin on the inner structure. Pectin-made beads showed a uniform and more compact inner structure with regard to alginate-based particles. Indeed, KL crystals resulted effectively included in the pectin matrix, whereas, for alginate beads, they resulted being distributed on the external layer (**Figure 7**). This effect may be due to the formation of several intermolecular hydrogen bonds and hydrophobic interactions between KL and pectin amino residues able to deeply stabilize the egg-box structure [61, 62]. The strong hydrogel network can determine a high shrinkage of the volume after drying process, leading to a significant reduction in mean diameter of the beads.

Results of dissolution tests (**Figure 8**) revealed that all KL-alginate beads provided fast and complete drug release in acidic medium, without any lag time, in 120 min. On the contrary, all pectin-based beads were able to achieve KL sustained release. The specific drug release profile from each formulations' series perfectly matches with beads morphology and structure data obtained by SEM investigation. The faster release of KL-alginate beads in SGF was related to KL crystals on the particle's surface and to the higher permeability of alginate matrix. Instead, Zn-pectinate beads showed a reduced swelling and erosion process in gastric environment as effect of their more compact texture [53, 63]. These data are consistent with recent literature studies, confirming the higher suitability of ALM-pectin to produce xerogel beads with improved technological properties compared to alginate [64, 65].

To improve delayed and sustained release performances, BKL_5 was selected as starting material for the preparation of a drug delivery platform made up by DR® capsules and BKL_5 (BKL_5/DR caps). Although gelatin capsules disaggregate after few minutes in simulated biological

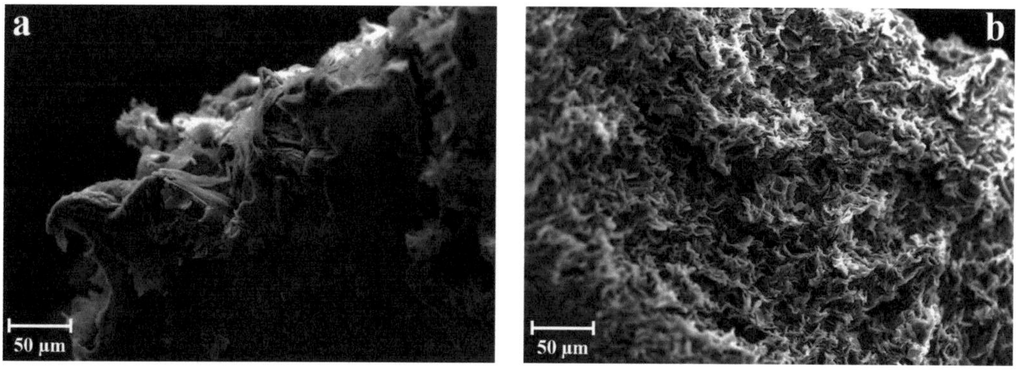

Figure 7. SEM microphotographs of cryo-fractured xerogel beads: (a) AKL_5 and (b) BK_5.

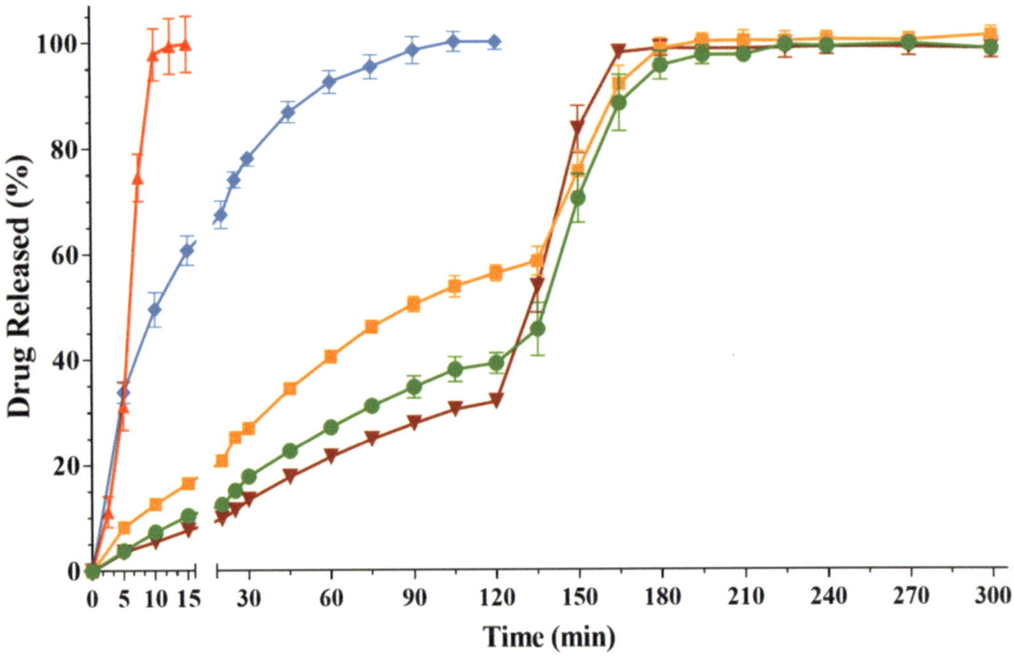

Figure 8. KL release profiles of formulations AKL_5 (-◆-), BKL_20 (-■-), BKL_10 (-●-), and BKL_5 (-▼-) compared to KL raw material (-▲-).

fluids, the selected capsules (DR®) can prolong the disaggregation step up to 75–90 min delaying the hydration process of BKL_5 beads in SGF. The optimized platform (BKL_5/DR caps) significantly reduced KL dissolution in SGF and showed a slower release in intestinal environment (**Figure 9**). This platform reduced KL release in SGF from 31.9 to 8.8% and prolonged its release in intestinal simulated fluid until 4.5 h (t=270 min) compared to 1 h (t=180 min) as observed for BKL_5. Only after the disaggregation of the capsule's body, beads are exposed to dissolution medium, starting later the dissolution process.

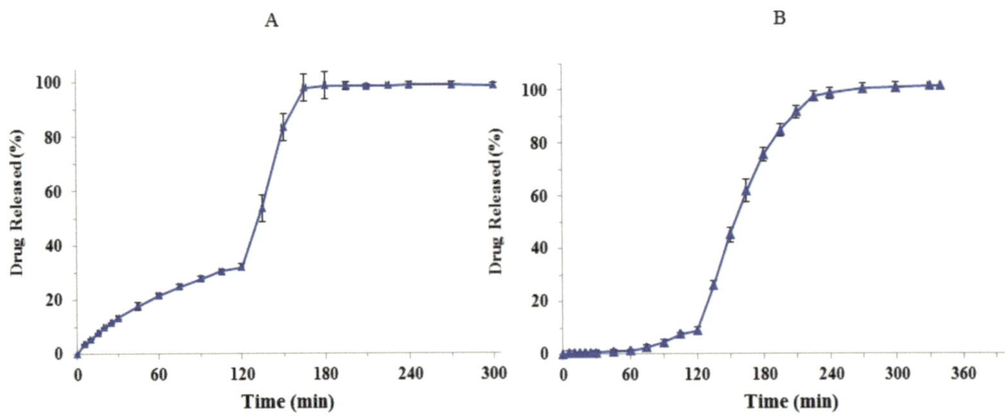

Figure 9. KL release profiles of BKL_5 (A) compared to the optimized platform BKL_5/DR caps (B).

Platform BKL_5 /DR caps may be potentially useful for the oral administration of highly soluble NSAIDs such as ketoprofen lysinate in the chronoterapeutic treatment of EMPs.

2.1.3. *Piroxicam-loaded core/shell beads as new ChDDS: design and characterization*

Piroxicam (PRX) is a NSAID of the oxicam class largely used to treat EMPs. PRX is included in the class II of the Biopharmaceutical Classification System as ketoprofen; however, it possesses different physical–chemical properties such as higher melting point and ampholytic nature. Thus, it may exist in different ionic forms at physiological pH [66]. PRX is rapidly and completely absorbed following oral administration (recommended dose in adults is 20 mg daily) and exhibits a long half-life (24-48h). However, its elimination is impaired in some elderly people [67], who represent the majority of patients affected by rheumatic diseases, resulting in a high inter-individual variability in the steady state plasma levels. Therefore, sustained release dosage forms capable of steady release of PRX over prolonged periods may overcome such variability due to erratic drug elimination [68].

In the case of PRX, we investigated the possibility to develop multiparticulate beads based on a blend of natural polysaccharides (monolayered particles) or a combination of polysaccharides with other polymers (double-layered particles). As discussed, beads based on single polysaccharide matrix may exhibit a premature release of the drug in the upper part of the GIT, making necessary the use of additional technological actions such as an enteric coating [53] or an envelopment in capsular devices [58]. However, a gel-matrix based on the combination of two or more polymers may be very effective [69].

2.1.3.1. *Methods*

Two series of piroxicam-loaded particles were produced using pectin/alginate (B/A) blends or pectin alone as carrier material. Several formulations were designed varying polymer total concentration between 4.0 and 6.0% (w/w), pectin alginate ratio from 10:0 to 10:2 and setting drug/polymers ratio at 1:20 (PRX_20) or 1:15 (PRX_15). Other operative conditions were set accordingly to previous experiments in order to obtain spherical hydrated beads with tough polymer matrix, smooth, and regular surface [69]. Beads micromeritics, solid state, and drug release properties were studied using established method (SEM, DSC, USP 36 Paddle Dissolution).

2.1.3.2. *Results and discussion*

High encapsulation efficiency (EE ranging from 62 to 93%), correlated to the increase of the polymer concentration in the feed, was achieved especially for BPRX_20, formulated with pectin alone. SEM analyses (**Figure 10**) highlighted that no crystals of piroxicam were visible on the surface, suggesting the drug complete entrapment within the polymeric matrix. Good micromeritics and encapsulation efficiency proposed the pectin-based formulation BPRX_20 as a starting point to develop a more efficient technological platform applying the two step core–shell approach previously tested for ketoprofen.

Beads BPRX_20 were coated by immersion with Eudragit® S100 to obtain an enteric coating able to avoid the erosion of the core pectin matrix and protect the drug in acidic medium [69].

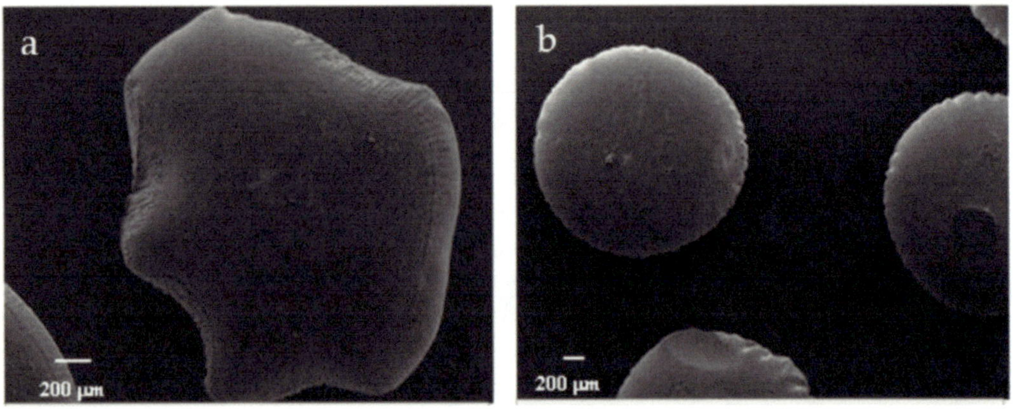

Figure 10. SEM microphotographs of pectin/alginate (a) and pectin beads (b) loaded with PRX produced by prilling and dried at room conditions.

Core/shell beads BPRX_20/E40 showed a drug release profile typical of gastro-resistant oral dosage forms, releasing less than 20% of piroxicam in SGF. In SIF, this formulation released approximately 50% of the loaded drug after 1 h achieving complete PRX release in approximately 5 h (**Figure 11**).

On the basis of these results, we can conclude that prilling technique in combination with an enteric coating is a very promising and simple two-step method to formulate core/shell beads as chronotherapeutic agents.

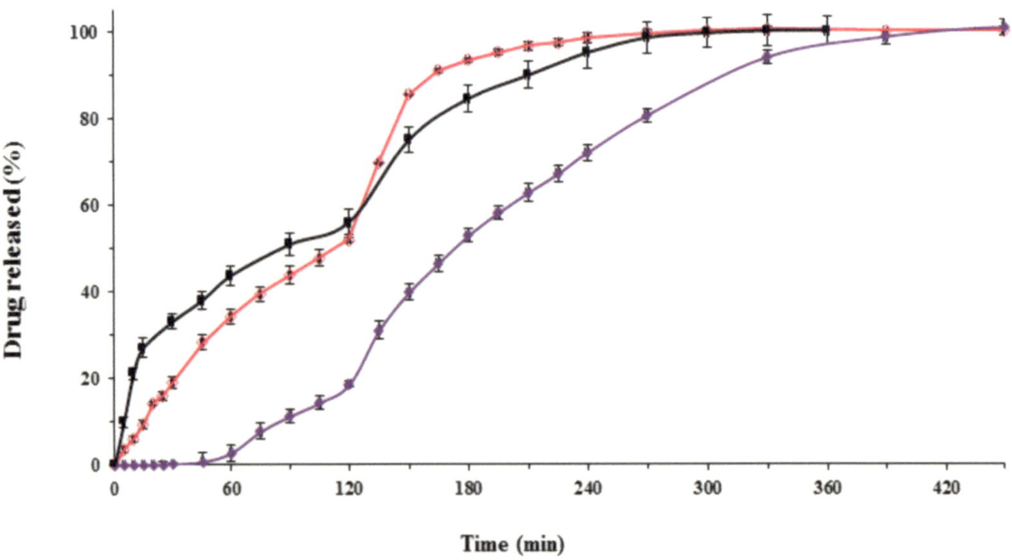

Figure 11. Release profiles of uncoated BPRX_20 (◇) and Eudragit®-coated beads formulations BPRX_20 _40 (◆), with regard to pure piroxicam (▪). Mean ± SD; (n=6).

Core–shell particles may also be obtained using a novel single step approach based on co-axial prilling technique. Core–shell systems composed of alginate (A) in the outer layer and pectin/piroxicam (B/PRX) as core were designed [70]. This innovative method employs multiple concentric nozzles to produce a smooth coaxial jet comprising polymer annular shell and core material, which are broken up by acoustic excitation into uniform core–shell droplets and gelled into a cross-linking solution. Alginate and pectin/PRX suspensions were pumped out through coxial nozzles with inner and outer diameters of 400 and 600 μm, respectively. Using volumetric flow rate of 10 ml/min, vibration frequency of 350 Hz and 100% amplitude of the vibration, the two viscous polymers suspensions subjected to prilling immediately formed droplets, which were dripped in a gelling Zn^{2+} bulk (Zn^{2+} concentration 10% w/v, pH 1.5 and cross-linking time 8 min). Schematic illustration of the core–shell process is shown in **Figure 12**.

Results showed that satisfying encapsulation efficiency values were obtained for the produced formulations (EE 58–93%). However, it is interesting to point out that EE for coated beads was related to shell integrity. In fact, formulation A/B_PRX10 (core/shell ratio 4:1 and PRX/pectin ratio 1:10) showing the most homogeneous coating presented very high EE (86.3%). The formation of complete alginate shell was able to prevent the piroxicam leaking from the droplets into the gelling medium during the polymer cross-linking phase; accordingly, a better entrapping of the drug within the core was obtained. The critical factor to obtain beads with regular shell was found to be the ratio between the nozzle viscosity of inner and outer polymer solutions (μ_c/μ_s). In fact, when nozzle viscosities ratio was less than 4, particles showed

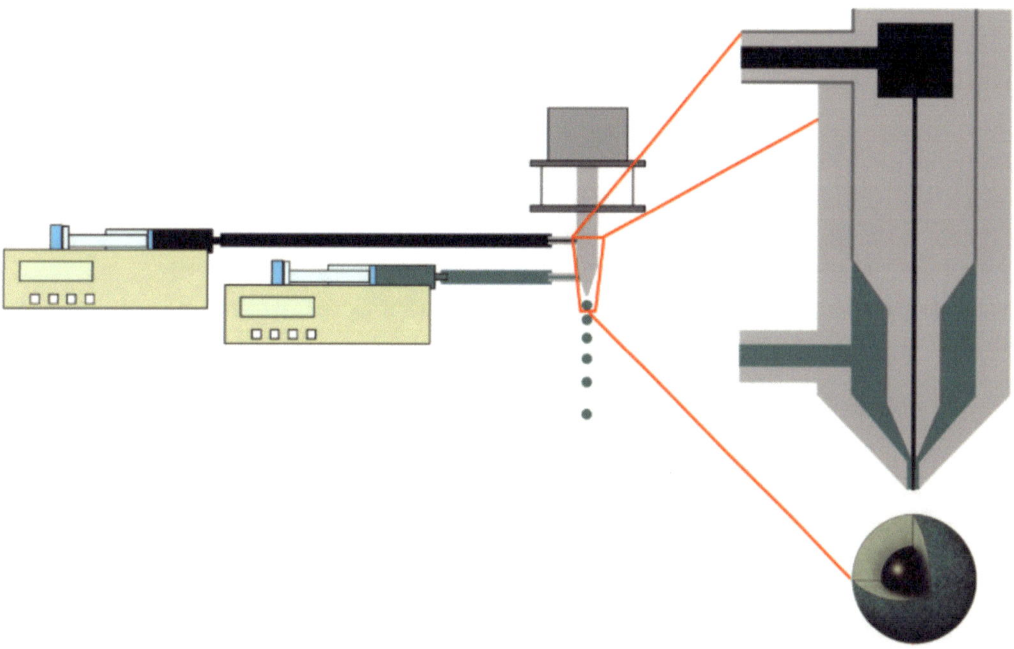

Figure 12. Schematic reproduction of prilling technology in coaxial configuration.

irregular or uncompleted alginate coating around the pectin core, whereas values over six matched with completely layered beads. During the droplet formation, the outer solution must be able to completely enclose the inner one. Therefore, the decrease in the alginate concentration and, subsequently, the decrease in the nozzle viscosity determine a regular core/shell beads formation [71].

To better understand the influence of drug content on polymeric matrix, cryofractured beads were also analyzed by fluorescent microscopy (FM). FM images of PRX-loaded pectin beads exhibited fluorescent spots due to crystals of piroxicam homogeneously encapsulated within the Zn-pectinate matrix (**Figure 13a–c**). FM analysis also proved that PRX core/shell beads, with B/A mass ratio of 4:1, presented the most homogeneous coating and, interestingly, showed that drug was confined into the particle inner matrix without any leaching into the alginate shell.

As reported elsewhere, Refs. [72–74] monolayered pectin beads act as a fast release formulation delivering approximately 50% of PRX in simulated gastric fluid and allowing the total drug release in SIF, after pH change, in approximately 2 h (**Figure 14**). On the contrary, core shell beads A/B_PRX10 release approximately 30% of PRX in SGF, achieving 100% in 5 h. The alginate shell decreases the initial burst effect, delaying both particles dissolution and drug diffusion in the simulated gastric fluid.

This study demonstrated that co-axial prilling technique can be used as a novel single-step approach for the manufacturing of core–shell particles containing NSAIDs. The most critical process parameter to obtain uniform double-layered particles was identified in the ratio between

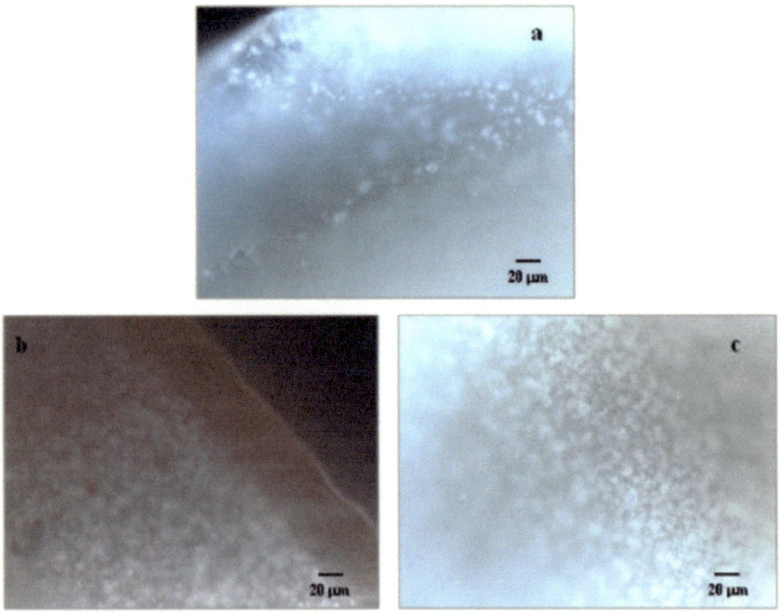

Figure 13. Fluorescent microscopy pictures of cryofractured PRX-loaded formulations: (a) uncoated Pct beads and (b and c) B/A beads.

http://dx.doi.org/10.5772/intechopen.68240

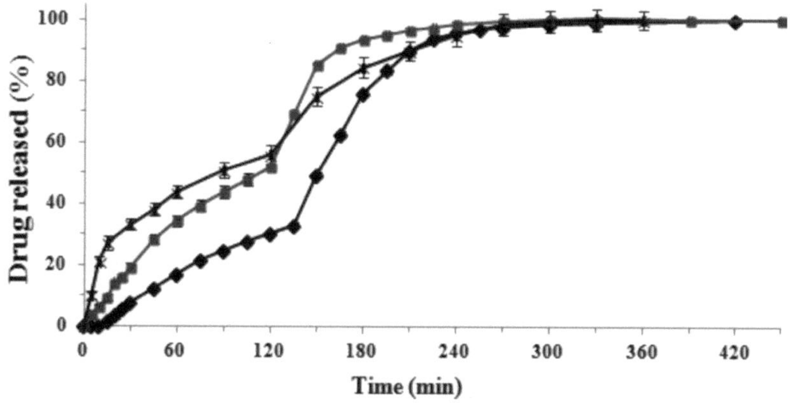

Figure 14. Release profiles of PRX raw material (-*-), monolayered pectin beads (-■-) and core/shell beads A/B_PRX10 (-◆-), performed using a pH change assay. Mean ± SD (n = 6).

inner and outer solution viscosities. The optimized core/shell (A/B_PRX10) beads can be considered either as a self-consistent dosage form or as a formulation to be hosted in suitable gastro-resistant capsule with the aim to further delay drug release meeting the requirements of EMPs.

2.2. Prilling in tandem with microwave-assisted drying

Hydrogel drying can also be conducted using alternative methods to conventional techniques. Each drying process has a different impact on structural characteristics of the dried beads especially on release properties. Particularly, in recent years, microwaves (MW) assisted heating has gained great interest in many applications with special reference to pharmaceutical processing. Several benefits can be obtained from technologies such as short processing time, better products uniformity and yields, energy saving, reduced production costs, as well as the ability to confer unique structural characteristics to the end materials. Recently, MW heating technology has been shown to be useful in the design of single-unit dosage forms such as solid dispersion, granules, and tablets [75–78]. Moreover, in the case of dextran-based formulations (i.e., alginate, pectin, and chitosan), MW irradiation leads to obtain xerogels with modified drug release properties due to the extent of polymer cross-linking and drug-excipient complexation [79, 80].

The efficiency of MW-assisted drying process is strongly influenced by dielectric, thermal, and other physical properties, as well as by moisture content of the irradiated material [81–84]. Under the influence of microwaves, the highly polarizable H_2O molecules can rotate rapidly in an attempt to align themselves with the alternating field, determining the frictional heat that promotes water evaporation. This forms the basis of microwave-assisted drying.

In view of these considerations, it is expected that MW heating is suitable to dry dissipative materials as carbohydrate-based hydrated beads manufactured by prilling. Therefore, the feasibility of joining prilling and MW-assisted treatments as a tandem technique was investigated to produce alginate-based xerogels with tailored NSAIDs release. Particularly, in this case, we selected two NSAIDs: ketoprofen (K) and piroxicam (PRX).

2.2.1. Release characteristics of ketoprofen-loaded beads obtained by prilling-dielectric treatments

As described by Auriemma et al. ketoprofen-loaded beads were obtained using prilling in tandem with dielectric treatments [85].

2.2.1.1. Materials and methods

Hydrated beads loaded with ketoprofen were manufactured by prilling and dried using MW-assisted heating under different radiation conditions (MW, power level I–IV) as control beads dried by air-bulk heating (tray oven) at 105°C and air-bulk room conditions were prepared. During the research, we studied the effects of different MW irradiation levels on particles micromeritics (i.e., morphology, size distribution, matrix porosity, and solid state of the loaded drug) and drug release behavior using established method (SEM, DSC, USP 36 Paddle Dissolution).

2.2.1.2. Results and discussion

Drug content and encapsulation efficiency were not influenced by the drying method. Particularly, ADC increased from 8 to 25% in accordance with the increasing of drug/polymer ratio (1:10 up to 1:3), and EE was remarkably high (over 93%) without any variation due to the drying process. In addition, as shown in **Figure 15**, the regime of MW irradiation had an important role on drying curves. MW irradiation process conducted at levels IV and III showed a drying rate essentially superimposable in the first 15 min. This might be due to the penetrative and volumetric heating nature of microwaves interesting the water migration from the inside out of the particles [86]. On the contrary, weaker irradiations needed prolonged times to eliminate water from particles. Conventional heating methods require, instead, even more prolonged process times (12–18 h at room conditions and 7 h for tray oven). This effect is probably due to the high thermal capacity and the low thermal diffusivity of hydrated beads.

Morphological analysis showed main differences in particle mean diameters for beads dried at different regime of MW irradiation. In fact, beads dried in MW continuous regime (level IV) exhibited the highest mean diameter (around 1.4 mm), while beads exposed to the weakest irradiation (level I) presented the lowest mean diameter (1.3 mm). Surface roughness as well as the number of cracks and craters on beads surface increased when level IV MW regime was used as shown by SEM analysis (**Figure 16b**, **c**).

Moreover, ketoprofen was in the amorphous state when drying was conducted at MW level IV due to the harsh regime of irradiation [87], whereas only few crystals without any trace of amorphous drug on the particle surface were observed for MW level II dried beads, as confirmed by X-ray analysis (**Figure 17**).

Regarding release properties, dielectric treatments provided a modulation of drug release (**Figure 18**). While beads dried at room conditions showed the typical behavior of enteric formulations, MW-treated beads at level IV acted as a conventional release formulation exhibiting a fast drug release without any lag time. In this case, the presence of solid ketoprofen and cracks on the bead surface (SEM images in **Figure 16**) allow an immediate release of the drug (45–50% in SGF) and a faster and continuous penetration of the dissolution medium inside the

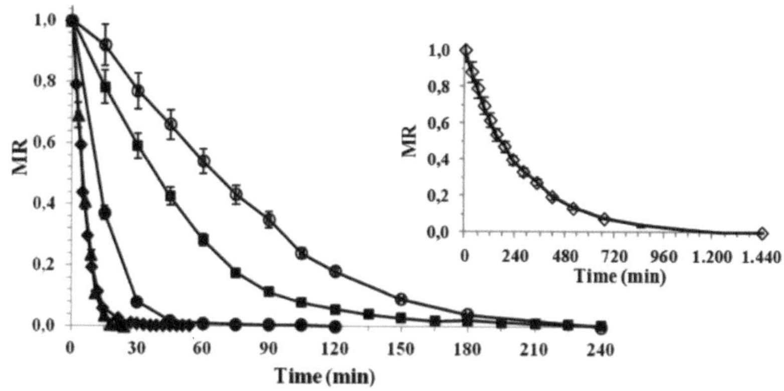

Figure 15. Drying curves of ketoprofen-loaded beads produced with 1.75% (w/w) alginate solution dried at different microwave irradiation levels: IV (-▲-); III (-◆-); II (-●-); I (-■-); tray oven drying at 105°C (–o–) and room conditions drying (-▲-) are also reported. Mean ± SD; (n=6).

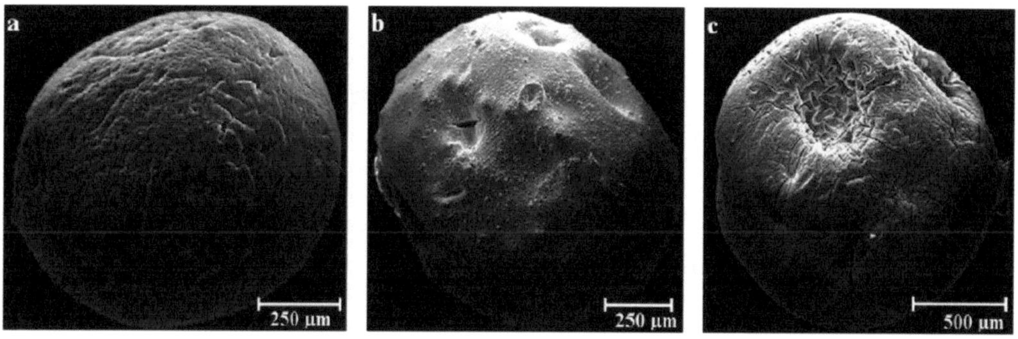

Figure 16. SEM microphotographs of K-loaded alginate beads dried in different conditions: (a) at room conditions, (b) level I, and (c) level IV microwave irradiation.

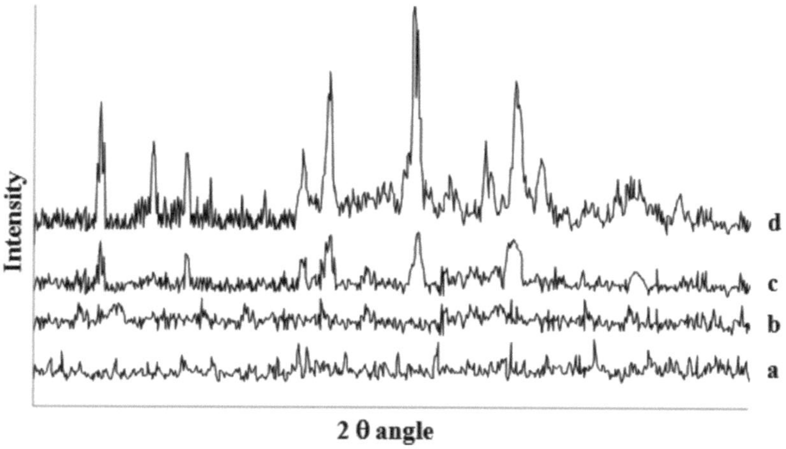

Figure 17. (a) X-ray diffraction patterns of blank alginate beads; K-loaded alginate bead treated at different microwave power levels: (b) IV; (c) III; and (d) pure crystalline ketoprofen.

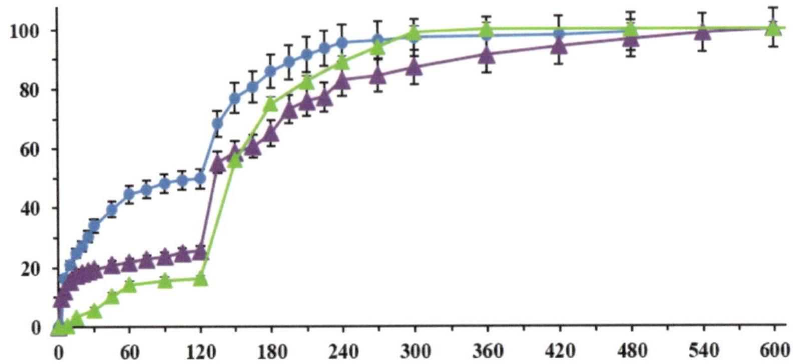

Figure 18. Release profiles of dried beads formulated with 1.75% (w/w) alginate solution and loaded with ketoprofen 8% (w/w) dried at room temperature (-▲-) and by MW treatments at: level I (-▲-) and level IV (-●-). Mean ± SD; (n=6).

alginate matrix in both SGF and SIF (complete release in about 2 h in SIF). A different behavior was observed for beads exposed to MW at level I. Drug release was significantly reduced in SGF, whereas it was prolonged and sustained until 6 h in SIF, as shown in **Figure 18**. The non-porous matrix and the structure integrity of the dried beads obtained with level I irradiation seem able to protect the drug in acidic medium and to achieve a prolonged/sustained release of ketoprofen in SIF, probably due to the interaction between drug and polymer matrix promoted by MW irradiation at level I [79].

2.2.2. *Release characteristics of piroxicam-loaded beads obtained by prilling-dielectric treatments*

Comparable results were obtained applying prilling/MW tandem technique to produce alginate beads loaded with piroxicam.

2.2.2.1. *Results and discussion*

Overall results from particles' technological analysis showed high values of encapsulation efficiency (over 85%) and a very narrow dimensional distribution.

SEM analyses showed that MW at levels III-IV drying process led to beads with small spots of crystalline piroxicam coming out of the surface (**Figure 19b** and **c**), whereas unspotted surface was obtained by MW irradiation at level I (**Figure 19a**). As reported in the literature, amorphous piroxicam shows a strong tendency to crystallize in either cubic (β) or needle form (α) [88]. The highest level of irradiation (MW level IV) allowed to obtain only the cubic form of crystalline PRX (**Figure 19c**). However, when MW level III was applied, both polymorphs (β cubic and α needle forms) were identified (**Figure 19b**).

Results of dissolution tests showed that the highest MW level (IV) produced a piroxicam intestinal dosage form with total PRX liberation in less than 1 h in simulated intestinal fluid. On the contrary, the lowest MW level (I) allowed to obtain a more sustained drug release profile (**Figure 20**). Differently from alginate/ketoprofen beads, where the presence of the drug (in amorphous or crystalline state) on the bead surface affected the release rate [85], in this case, drug release was not influenced by cubic or needle crystalline forms.

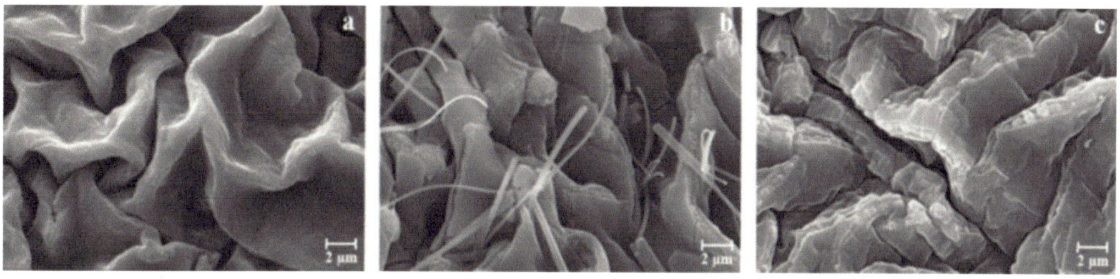

Figure 19. SEM microphotographs of beads' surface (alginate 1.75% w/w; PRX 7% w/w) after MW irradiation at level I (a), III (b), and IV (c).

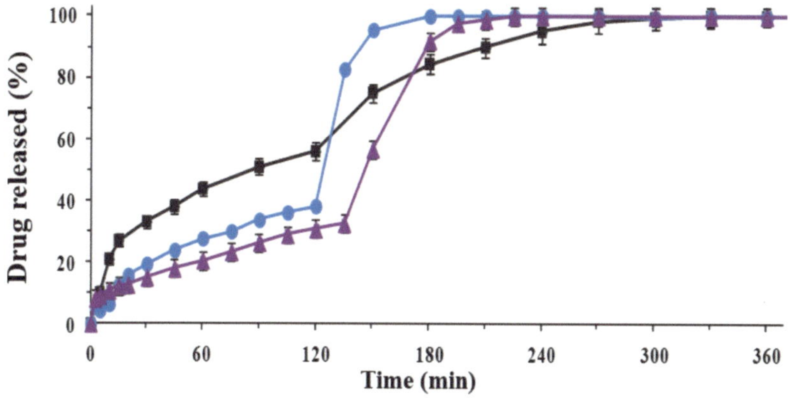

Figure 20. Drug release profile of piroxicam-loaded beads (alginate 1.75% w/w and PRX 7% w/w) dried by MW at level I (-▲-) and level IV (-●-) compared to piroxicam raw material (-■-). Mean±S.D. (n = 6).

The obtained results suggest that surface and inner characteristics of the alginate/piroxicam beads (roughness, network of cracks, and a fraction of crystalline piroxicam on beads surface) are strongly able to modulate the drug dissolution.

On the basis of these results, we can state that prilling/MW tandem technique can be used as a simple method to formulate alginate beads with tailored NSAIDs release depending on drug characteristics and MW irradiation level. Dielectric treatments compared to conventional methods offer several advantages such as faster drying kinetics leading to energy saving with low-operative costs and the possibility to modulate drug release and dissolution profiles without affecting drug loading.

2.3. Prilling in tandem with supercritical fluid-assisted drying

Another approach to develop dried beads with modified drug release behavior is represented by the use of prilling technique in tandem with supercritical fluids. Supercritical drying processing has also gained wide acceptance as an alternative to conventional drying techniques. Particularly, supercritical antisolvent extraction (SAE) overcomes the problems encountered with traditional drying methods and may preserve the nanoporous structure of the wet gel-beads leading to aerogels. Among the many possible supercritical fluids (SFs), carbon dioxide

(CO_2) is the most widely used. It has readily accessible critical points and as a process solvent offers the additional benefits of being nontoxic, nonflammable, environmentally acceptable, inexpensive, and can be used at a mild critical temperature suitable for processing thermally labile compounds. One major challenge for the preparation of alginate-based aerogels is to eliminate the liquid solvent from the gel, while avoiding the collapse of the already existing nanoporous structure with the subsequent shrinkage of the dried gel. Supercritical CO_2-assisted drying is the most appropriate drying technique able to overcome these problems [89]. However, SC-CO_2 shows only a very limited affinity with water; therefore, in principle water-based solution cannot be treated. Aerogel production technology comprises a series of steps such as formation of a polysaccharide water solution (hydrogel), gelation of the sol induced by cross-linking promoters, replacement of water by a solvent (usually ethanol or acetone) and, finally, solvent elimination [90]. Various aerogel forms (monolithical cylinders, spheres, membranes, tubes, etc) may be produced by different techniques (moulding, extrusion, and milling); however, beads are preferred for applications in pharmaceutics.

2.3.1. *Ketoprofen-loaded aerogel beads produced by tandem prilling/SAE*

Recently, we designed and developed alginate-based aerogel beads by using prilling in combination with SC-CO_2 processing [73]. As above mentioned, water-based "materials" cannot be dried directly with SC-CO_2 due to the low solubility of water in the supercritical phase. To overcome this limitation, we tested either gelling process in alcoholic solution or solvent exchange pretreatment of hydrate beads to allow successful elimination of the solvent and to obtain aerogel formation. For this study, ketoprofen (K) was used as a model drug. Beads were produced by prilling and cross-linked by calcium cations either in ethanol (sol → alcogels) or in aqueous solutions (sol → hydrogels). In the latter case, solvent exchange was necessary to replace water by ethanol obtaining alcogels that were successively subjected to solvent extraction by SC-CO_2 leading to aerogels. Aerogel beads were designed to obtain a prompt release of the loaded drug and, consequently, a rapid onset of the analgesic effect, as required in postoperative pain [91, 92], dental surgery [93], renal and ureteral acute colic [94, 95].

2.3.1.1. *Methods*

Two series of beads were manufactured using 0.3 M $CaCl_2$ in water or in ethanol as cross-linker solutions. All hydrated beads showed spherical shape (SC, 0.98 ± 0.01), smooth and regular surface and a mean diameter ranging between 3.81 and 3.97 mm. Tiny white solid spots were present inside all loaded particles, whereas unloaded beads were almost transparent. Supercritical CO_2 drying was performed by SAE laboratory apparatus at 150 bar and 37°C.

2.3.1.2. *Results and discussion*

In the selected drying conditions, reduced particle shrinkage was observed and the internal porous texture of the parent hydrogel was preserved, as illustrated in the SEM image (**Figure 21**), where the nanofibrous alginate network is well visible. SC-CO_2 drying determined a reduction of beads diameters ranging between 2.70 and 3.11 mm. As a comparison, drying process was also conducted using a homogenous amount of hydrated beads exposed

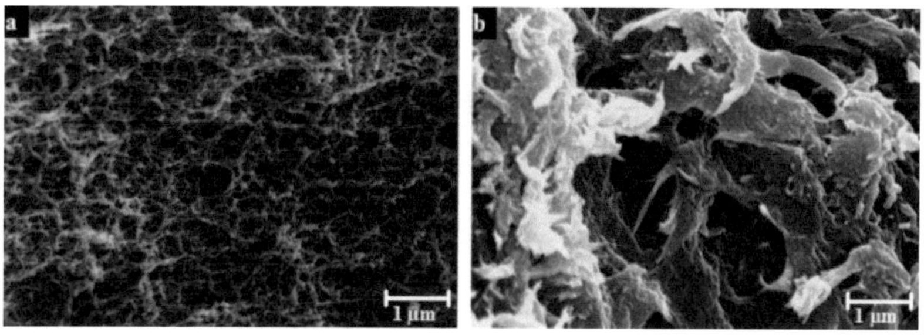

Figure 21. SEM microphotographs of ketoprofen-loaded alginate beads inner matrix dried using different processes: supercritical CO_2 treatment (a) and room conditions (b).

to room conditions and, alternatively, to air-bulk heating (tray oven) at 105°C. As expected, both convective processing methods took long times (tray oven 4- h; room conditions 12–18 h). Moreover, an extensive volume shrinkage was observed when convective drying methods were used (diameter 1.8 mm with SD lower than 3%) due to the collapse of the polymer matrix during the slow solvent evaporation.

Encapsulation efficiency values were greater for beads subjected to conventional drying than for those treated with supercritical carbon dioxide without relevant differences between room conditions and tray oven. As previously reported, the transport phenomena involved in the supercritical fluid extraction may cause the extraction of small quantities of drug [96]; this effect may explain the observed decrease in EE. In detail, convective dried beads exhibited EE around 52 or 94% depending on ethanol or aqueous cross-linking, respectively. In the same gelling conditions, SC-CO_2–treated beads showed EE around 6 or 59%.

The inner matrix structure was deeply influenced by different drying techniques. Supercritical treatment produced a nanoporous alginate matrix characterized by a network of nanopores with diameters around 200 nm. Convective drying leads to a compact matrix with less and larger pores where the nanofibrous structure was completely lost, as shown in **Figure 21b**. It is well known that one of the major challenges in aerogel production from hydrogels is the solvent elimination that must occur without inducing the collapse of the porous structure; in this regard, the fast elimination of ethanol from alcogels by SC-CO_2 processing is able to prevent the collapsing of the parent gel structure [97, 98].

More interestingly, the procedure for producing the alcogel-influenced habitus of solid K into the inner matrix, as shown by SEM images (**Figure 22**) of cryo-fractured dried particles. Cross-linking alginate in ethanol (**Figure 22a**) leads to crystal clusters of K drug embedded into the aerogel, beads from aqueous cross-linking, and water replacement by ethanol (**Figure 22b**) showed only nanometric particles of amorphous K.

The dissolution profile of K from SC-CO_2–treated beads (**Figure 23**) presented an enhanced burst effect in SGF (more than 75% of the encapsulated drug in 30 min in acidic medium) for aerogels obtained cross-linking the particles in aqueous $CaCl_2$ and then replacing water with ethanol. Formulations cross-linked in ethanol as well as crystalline material released less than 40% of K in the same time. The considerable increase of the drug dissolution rate for

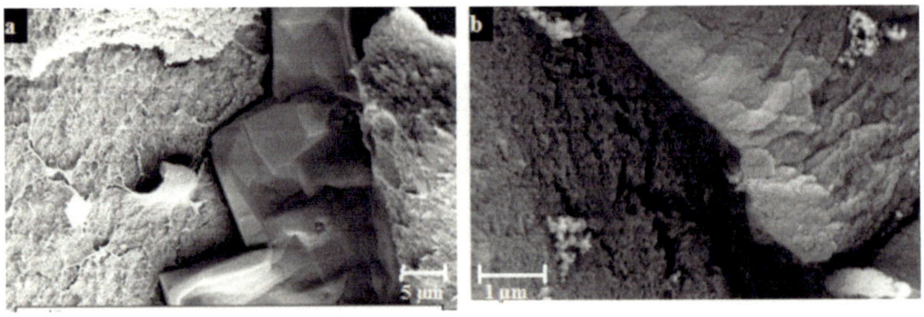

Figure 22. SEM microphotographs of cryo-fractured ketoprofen-loaded alginate beads dried by supercritical CO_2 previously cross-linked in ethanol (a) or water (b).

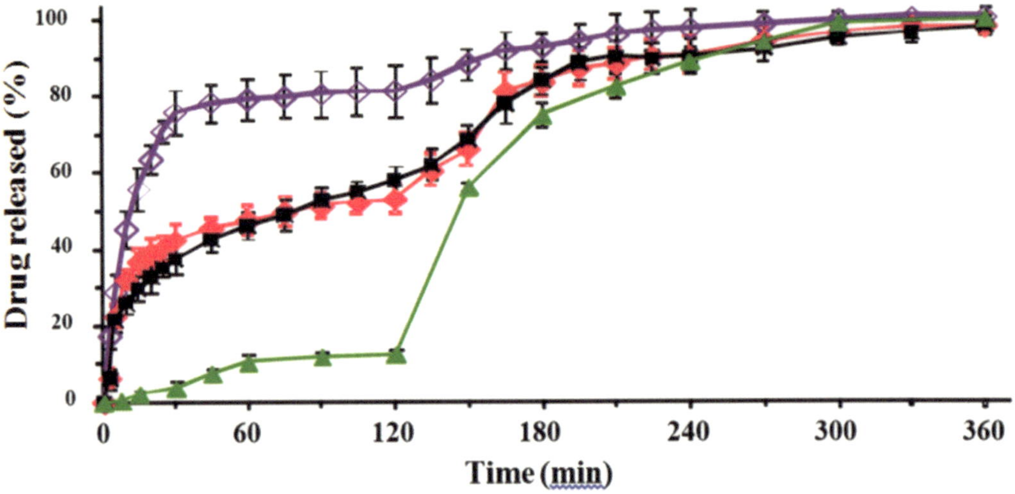

Figure 23. Release profiles of K-loaded alginate beads dried by SC-CO_2 treatment previously cross-linked in ethanol (-◆-) or water (-◇-), exposed to room conditions (-▲-) in comparison to pure ketoprofen (-■-). Mean ± SD; (n=6).

formulations cross-linked in water can be explained by the high porosity of the aerogel and by the increased surface-volume ratio due to nanometric dimensions of the solid amorphous ketoprofen [99] embedded into the nanoporous structure.

In conclusion, prilling process in tandem with SC-CO_2-assisted drying allows to produce alginate-based aerogel. Drug loading capacity and encapsulation efficiency reached approximately 59%. Interestingly, after SC-CO_2 drying, particles keep constant spherical shape and narrow dimensional range and retain the porosity of the parent hydrated gel-matrix. The highly nanoporous drug carrier with high surface area provides enhanced and controlled fast release of ketoprofen. Formulations cross-linked in water, and then replacing water with ethanol, improve significantly the dissolution rate of K, especially in simulated gastric fluid. High enhancement of the drug dissolution can be very useful in favoring drug liberation and absorption in order to obtain a rapid onset of the therapeutic effect as required in acute inflammation. Alginate-based aerogel produced by prilling in combination with SC-CO_2–assisted drying may be proposed as fast dissolving formulation for slightly soluble NSAIDs belonging to BCS class II.

3. Conclusions

Particle engineering through prilling-based techniques can be applied to widely used NSAIDs as ketoprofen and piroxicam to develop new drug delivery systems, which meet current therapeutic input and health demands. This approach allows to fit specific therapeutic needs of inflammatory-based diseases. Particularly, prilling technique in tandem with dieletric treatment at high MW level or with supercritical (SC-CO_2) drying allows to produce porous microparticles with high surface area able to enhance the dissolution rate of slightly soluble NSAIDs (BCS class II). These systems providing a fast drug release may promote a rapid therapeutic effect after oral administration, as required in acute pain and inflammation. Instead, using prilling in combination with conventional or dielectric drying at low MW levels, it is possible to obtain engineered particles with slower NSAIDs release compared to conventional and commercially available formulations. By opportunely selecting carrier materials or gelling conditions or using additional technological actions such as enteric coating or capsular devices, it is possible to obtain chronotherapeutic drug delivery systems useful to treat EMPs. The potential benefits in chronotherapy of these systems were also confirmed using an *in vivo* model of inflammation. The control and strong delay of NSAIDs release make these drug products suitable to be taken at bed time and act in the early morning hours.

Author details

Giulia Auriemma[1]*, Andrea Cerciello[1,2] and Rita P. Aquino[1]

*Address all correspondence to: gauriemma@unisa.it

1 Department of Pharmacy, University of Salerno, Fisciano (SA), Italy

2 University of Salerno, Fisciano (SA), Italy

References

[1] Pivette P, Faivre V, Mancini L, Gueutin C, Daste G, Ollivon M, et al. Controlled release of a highly hydrophilic API from lipid microspheres obtained by prilling: Analysis of drug and water diffusion processes with X-ray-based methods. Journal of Controlled Release. 2012;**158**(3):393-402. http://dx.doi.org/10.1016/j.jconrel.2011.11.027

[2] Paolino D, Sinha P, Fresta M, Ferrari M. Drug Delivery Systems. J.G. Webster (Ed.), Encyclopedia of Medical Devices and Instrumentation. (2nd ed.), John Wiley & Sons, Inc.; 2006, pp. 437-495.

[3] Straub RH, Cutolo M. Circadian rhythms in rheumatoid arthritis: Implications for pathophysiology and therapeutic management. Arthritis & Rheumatism. 2007;**56**(2):399-408.

[4] Gibbs JE, Ray DW. The role of the circadian clock in rheumatoid arthritis. Arthritis Research & Therapy. 2013;**15**(1):1.

[5] Storms WW. Pharmacologic approaches to daytime and nighttime symptoms of allergic rhinitis. Journal of Allergy and Clinical Immunology. 2004;**114**(5 Suppl):S146-S53. Epub 2004/11/13. 10.1016/j.jaci.2004.08.045

[6] Ambedkar Sunil S, Venkata Srikanth M, Sreenivasa Rao N, Venkata Ramana Murthy K. Chronotherapeutic drug delivery from indomethacin compression coated tablets for early morning pain associated rheumatoid arthritis. Current Drug Delivery. 2013; **10**(1):109-121.

[7] Smith DH, Neutel JM, Weber MA. A new chronotherapeutic oral drug absorption system for verapamil optimizes blood pressure control in the morning. American Journal of Hypertension. 2001;**14**(1):14-19.

[8] Lemmer B. Circadian rhythms and drug delivery. Journal of Controlled Release. 1991;**16**(1-2):63-74. http://dx.doi.org/10.1016/0168-3659(91)90031-8

[9] Youan B-BC. Chronopharmaceutics: Gimmick or clinically relevant approach to drug delivery? Journal of Controlled Release. 2004;**98**(3):337-353. http://dx.doi.org/10.1016/j.jconrel.2004.05.015

[10] Lévi F, Okyar A. Circadian clocks and drug delivery systems: Impact and opportunities in chronotherapeutics. Expert Opinion on Drug Delivery. 2011;**8**(12):1535-1541.doi:10.1517/17425247.2011.618184

[11] Busetti C, Crimella T. Methods for treating early morning pathologies. Google Patents; 2006.

[12] Arvidson NG, Gudbjörnsson B, Elfman L, Rydén AC, Tötterman TH, Hällgren R. Circadian rhythm of serum interleukin-6 in rheumatoid arthritis. Annals of the Rheumatic Diseases. 1994;**53**(8):521-524.10.1136/ard.53.8.521

[13] Cutolo M. Glucocorticoids and chronotherapy in rheumatoid arthritis. RMD Open. 2016;**2**(1):e000203.

[14] Lotlikar V, Kedar U, Shidhaye S, Kadam V. pH-responsive dual pulse multiparticulate dosage form for treatment of rheumatoid arthritis. Drug Development and Industrial Pharmacy. 2010;**36**(11):1295-1302.

[15] Levi F, Louarn CL, Reinberg A. Timing optimizes sustained-release indomethacin treatment of osteoarthritis. Clinical Pharmacology & Therapeutics. 1985;**37**(1):77-84.

[16] Smolensky MH, Peppas NA. Chronobiology, drug delivery, and chronotherapeutics. Advanced Drug Delivery Reviews. 2007;**59**(9-10):828-851. DOI: http://dx.doi.org/10.1016/j.addr.2007.07.001

[17] Hermida RC, Ayala DE, Calvo C, Portaluppi F, Smolensky MH. Chronotherapy of hypertension: Administration-time-dependent effects of treatment on the circadian pattern of blood pressure. Advanced Drug Delivery Reviews. 2007;**59**(9-10):923-939. DOI: http://dx.doi.org/10.1016/j.addr.2006.09.021

[18] Cerciello A, Auriemma G, Morello S, Aquino RP, Del Gaudio P, Russo P. Prednisolone delivery platforms: Capsules and beads combination for a right timing therapy. PLoS One. 2016;**11**(7):e0160266. DOI: 10.1371/journal.pone.0160266

[19] Singh M, Hemant K, Ram M, Shivakumar H. Microencapsulation: A promising technique for controlled drug delivery. Research in Pharmaceutical Sciences. 2011;**5**(2):65-77.

[20] Dalmoro A, Barba AA, Lamberti G, d'Amore M. Intensifying the microencapsulation process: Ultrasonic atomization as an innovative approach. European Journal of Pharmaceutics and Biopharmaceutics. 2012;**80**(3):471-477. DOI: http://dx.doi.org/10.1016/j.ejpb.2012.01.006

[21] Del Gaudio P, Russo P, Rosaria Lauro M, Colombo P, Aquino R. Encapsulation of ketoprofen and ketoprofen lysinate by prilling for controlled drug release. AAPS PharmSciTech. 2009;**10**(4):1178-1185. DOI: 10.1208/s12249-009-9309-z

[22] Tran V-T, Benoît J-P, Venier-Julienne M-C. Why and how to prepare biodegradable, monodispersed, polymeric microparticles in the field of pharmacy? International Journal of Pharmaceutics. 2011;**407**(1):1-11.

[23] Berkland C, Kim K, Pack DW. Fabrication of PLG microspheres with precisely controlled and monodisperse size distributions. Journal of Controlled Release. 2001;**73**(1):59-74. DOI: http://dx.doi.org/10.1016/S0168-3659(01)00289-9

[24] Mazzitelli S, Tosi A, Balestra C, Nastruzzi C, Luca G, Mancuso F, et al. Production and characterization of alginate microcapsules produced by a vibrational encapsulation device. Journal of Biomaterials Applications. 2008; 23(2): 123-145.

[25] Zvonar A, Kristl J, KerÄ J, Grabnar PA. High celecoxib-loaded nanoparticles prepared by a vibrating nozzle device. Journal of Microencapsulation; 2009; 26(8): 748-759.

[26] Brandau E. US Patent No. 54726485; 1995.

[27] Dumas H, Tardy M, Rochat MH, Tayot JL. Prilling process applied to collagen solutions. Drug Development and Industrial Pharmacy. 1992;**18**(13):1395-1409.doi:10.3109/03639049209040847

[28] Kim I-Y, Seo S-J, Moon H-S, Yoo M-K, Park I-Y, Kim B-C, et al. Chitosan and its derivatives for tissue engineering applications. Biotechnology Advances. 2008;**26**(1):1-21. DOI: http://dx.doi.org/10.1016/j.biotechadv.2007.07.009

[29] Berkland C, Pack DW, Kim K. Microparticles. US Patent 6,669,961 B2; 2003.

[30] Brandenberger H, Widmer F. A new multinozzle encapsulation/immobilisation system to produce uniform beads of alginate. Journal of Biotechnology. 1998;**63**(1):73-80.

[31] Brandau T. Preparation of monodisperse controlled release microcapsules. International Journal of Pharmaceutics. 2002;**242**(1-2):179-184. DOI: http://dx.doi.org/10.1016/S0378-5173(02)00151-5

[32] DeRamos CM, Irwin AE, Nauss JL, Stout BE. ^{13}C NMR and molecular modeling studies of alginic acid binding with alkaline earth and lanthanide metal ions. Inorganica Chimica Acta. 1997;**256**(1):69-75. DOI: http://dx.doi.org/10.1016/S0020-1693(96)05418-7

[33] Braccini I, Grasso RP, Pérez S. Conformational and configurational features of acidic polysaccharides and their interactions with calcium ions: A molecular modeling investigation. Carbohydrate Research. 1999;**317**(1-4):119-130. DOPI: http://dx.doi.org/10.1016/S0008-6215(99)00062-2

[34] Hua S, Ma H, Li X, Yang H, Wang A. pH-sensitive sodium alginate/poly(vinyl alcohol) hydrogel beads prepared by combined Ca^{2+} crosslinking and freeze-thawing cycles for controlled release of diclofenac sodium. International Journal of Biological Macromolecules. 2010;**46**(5):517-523.

[35] Auriemma G. Prilling-based Tandem Techniques: Design and Development of NSAIDs Controlled Delivery Systems [thesis]. Fisciano: Universisy of Salerno; 2013.

[36] Zubizarreta L, Arenillas A, Domínguez A, Menéndez JA, Pis JJ. Development of microporous carbon xerogels by controlling synthesis conditions. Journal of Non-Crystalline Solids. 2008;**354**(10-11):817-825. DOI: http://dx.doi.org/10.1016/j.jnoncrysol.2007.08.015

[37] Léonard A, Job N, Blacher S, Pirard J-P, Crine M, Jomaa W. Suitability of convective air drying for the production of porous resorcinol–formaldehyde and carbon xerogels. Carbon. 2005;**43**(8):1808-1811. DOI: http://dx.doi.org/10.1016/j.carbon.2005.02.016

[38] Job N, Panariello F, Marien J, Crine M, Pirard J-P, Léonard A. Synthesis optimization of organic xerogels produced from convective air-drying of resorcinol–formaldehyde gels. Journal of Non-Crystalline Solids. 2006;**352**(1):24-34. DOI: http://dx.doi.org/10.1016/j.jnoncrysol.2005.11.024

[39] Menéndez JA, Juárez-Pérez EJ, Ruisánchez E, Calvo EG, Arenillas A. A microwave-based method for the synthesis of carbon xerogel spheres. Carbon. 2012;**50**(10):3555-3560. DOI: http://dx.doi.org/10.1016/j.carbon.2012.03.027

[40] Della Porta G, Del Gaudio P, De Cicco F, Aquino RP, Reverchon E. Supercritical drying of alginate beads for the development of aerogel biomaterials: Optimization of process parameters and exchange solvents. Industrial & Engineering Chemistry Research. 2013;**52**(34):12003-12009.

[41] Cerciello A, Auriemma G, Morello S, Pinto A, Del Gaudio P, Russo P, et al. Design and in vivo anti-inflammatory effect of ketoprofen delayed delivery systems. Journal of Pharmaceutical Sciences. 2015;**104**(10):3451-3458. Epub 2015/06/20.10.1002/jps.24554

[42] Cerciello A. Chronotherapeutic drug delivery in early morning pathologies: design and production of new NSAIDs/SAIDs polysaccharide-based systems [thesis]. 2017.

[43] Abbas SS, Schaalan MF, Bahgat AK, El-Denshary ES. Possible potentiation by certain antioxidants of the anti-inflammatory effects of diclofenac in rats. The Scientific World Journal. 2014;2014: 1-9.

[44] Gaweł M, Librowski T, Lipkowska A. Influence of zinc hydroaspartate on the anti-inflammatory and gastric activity of ketoprofen in rats. Pharmacological Reports. 2013; **65**(1):214-219.

[45] Yang L, Chu JS, Fix JA. Colon-specific drug delivery: New approaches and in vitro/in vivo evaluation. International Journal of Pharmaceutics. 2002;**235**(1):1-15.

[46] Rockville M. FDA Guidance for Industry: Extended release oral dosage forms: Development, evaluation and application of in vitro/in vivo correlation. 1997; BP2: 1-24.

[47] Wen H, Park K, editors. Oral Controlled Release Formulation Design and Drug Delivery: Theory to Practice. John Wiley & Sons; 2011; 364 p., DOI: 10.1002/9780470640487.

[48] Fotaki N. Flow-through cell apparatus (usp apparatus 4): Operation and features. Dissolution Technologies. 2011;**18**(4):46-49.

[49] Gao Z. In vitro dissolution testing with flow-through method: A technical note. AAPS PharmSciTech. 2009;**10**(4):1401-1405.

[50] Hu J, Kyad A, Ku V, Zhou P, Cauchon N. A comparison of dissolution testing on lipid soft gelatin capsules using USP apparatus 2 and apparatus 4. Dissolution Technologies. 2005;**12**(2):6-9.

[51] Medina JR, Salazar DK, Hurtado M, Cortes AR, Domínguez-Ramírez AM. Comparative in vitro dissolution study of carbamazepine immediate-release products using the USP paddles method and the flow-through cell system. Saudi Pharmaceutical Journal. 2014;**22**(2):141-147.

[52] Moogooee M, Ramezanzadeh H, Jasoori S, Omidi Y, Davaran S. Synthesis and in vitro studies of cross-linked hydrogel nanoparticles containing amoxicillin. Journal of Pharmaceutical Sciences. 2011;**100**(3):1057-1066.

[53] Cerciello A, Auriemma G, Del Gaudio P, Sansone F, Aquino RP, Russo P. A novel core–shell chronotherapeutic system for the oral administration of ketoprofen. Journal of Drug Delivery Science and Technology. 2016;**32**, Part B:126-131. DOI: http://dx.doi.org/10.1016/j.jddst.2015.07.017

[54] Assifaoui A, Loupiac C, Chambin O, Cayot P. Structure of calcium and zinc pectinate films investigated by FTIR spectroscopy. Carbohydrate Research. 2010;**345**(7):929-933.

[55] Sriamornsak P. Chemistry of pectin and its pharmaceutical uses: A review. Silpakorn University International Journal. 2003;**3**(1-2):206-228.

[56] Prajapati CV, Patel RP, Prajapati BG. Formulation, optimization and evaluation of sustained release microsphere of ketoprofen. Journal of Pharmacy and Bioallied Sciences. 2012;**4**(Suppl 1):0975-7406.

[57] Cimini A, Brandolini L, Gentile R, Cristiano L, Menghini P, Fidoamore A, et al. Gastroprotective effects of L-lysine salification of ketoprofen in ethanol-injured gastric mucosa. Journal of Cellular Physiology. 2015;**230**(4):813-820. Epub 2014/10/08.10.1002/jcp.24809

[58] Cerciello A, Auriemma G, Del Gaudio P, Cantarini M, Aquino RP. Natural polysaccharides platforms for oral controlled release of ketoprofen lysine salt. Drug Development and Industrial Pharmacy. 2016;**42**(12):2063-2069. Epub 2016/05/31.10.1080/03639045.2016.1195401

[59] Mesbahi G, Jamalian J, Farahnaky A. A comparative study on functional properties of beet and citrus pectins in food systems. Food Hydrocolloids. 2005;**19**(4):731-738. DOI: http://dx.doi.org/10.1016/j.foodhyd.2004.08.002

[60] Kim Y, Kim Y-S, Yoo S-H, Kim K-O. Molecular differences of low methoxy pectins induced by pectin methyl esterase I: Effects on texture, release and perception of aroma in gel systems. Food Chemistry. 2010;**123**(2):451-455. DOI: http://dx.doi.org/10.1016/j.foodchem.2010.04.067

[61] Liu L, Fishman ML, Hicks KB, Kende M. Interaction of various pectin formulations with porcine colonic tissues. Biomaterials. 2005;**26**(29):5907-5916. DOI: http://dx.doi.org/10.1016/j.biomaterials.2005.03.005

[62] Sato Y, Miyawaki O. Analysis of intermolecular interaction among pectin molecules in aqueous sugar solutions. Food Science and Technology Research. 2008;**14**(3):232-238.

[63] Pal K, Singh VK, Anis A, Thakur G, Bhattacharya MK. Hydrogel-based controlled release formulations: Designing considerations, characterization techniques and applications. Polymer-Plastics Technology and Engineering. 2013;**52**(14):1391-422.

[64] Belscak-Cvitanovic A, Komes D, Karlovic S, Djakovic S, Spoljaric I, Mrsic G, et al. Improving the controlled delivery formulations of caffeine in alginate hydrogel beads combined with pectin, carrageenan, chitosan and psyllium. Food Chemistry. 2015;**167**: 378-386.

[65] Voo WP, Ravindra P, Tey BT, Chan ES. Comparison of alginate and pectin based beads for production of poultry probiotic cells. Journal of Bioscience and Bioengineering. 2011;**111**(3):294-299.

[66] Geckle JM, Rescek DM, Whipple EB. Zwitterionic piroxicam in polar solution. Magnetic Resonance in Chemistry. 1989;**27**(2):150-154. DOI: 10.1002/mrc.1260270211

[67] Verbeeck R, Richardson C, Blocka K. Clinical pharmacokinetics of piroxicam. Journal of Rheumatology. 1986;**13**(4):789-796.

[68] Joseph NJ, Lakshmi S, Jayakrishnan A. A floating-type oral dosage form for piroxicam based on hollow polycarbonate microspheres: In vitro and in vivo evaluation in rabbits. Journal of Controlled Release. 2002;**79**(1-3):71-79. Epub 2002/02/21.

[69] Auriemma G, Mencherini T, Russo P, Stigliani M, Aquino RP, Del Gaudio P. Prilling for the development of multi-particulate colon drug delivery systems: Pectin vs. pectin–alginate beads. Carbohydrate Polymers. 2013;**92**(1):367-373. DOI: http://dx.doi.org/10.1016/j.carbpol.2012.09.056

[70] Del Gaudio P, Auriemma G, Russo P, Mencherini T, Campiglia P, Stigliani M, et al. Novel co-axial prilling technique for the development of core–shell particles as delayed drug delivery systems. European Journal of Pharmaceutics and Biopharmaceutics. 2014;**87**(3):541-547. DOI: http://dx.doi.org/10.1016/j.ejpb.2014.02.010

[71] Routh AF, Russel WB. A process model for latex film formation:? Limiting regimes for individual driving forces. Langmuir. 1999;**15**(22):7762-7773.10.1021/la9903090

[72] Bourgeois S, Laham A, Besnard M, Andremont A, Fattal E. In vitro and in vivo evaluation of pectin beads for the colon delivery of β-lactamases. Journal of Drug Targeting. 2005;**13**(5):277-284. DOI: 10.1080/10611860500206583

[73] Del Gaudio P, Auriemma G, Mencherini T, Porta GD, Reverchon E, Aquino RP. Design of alginate-based aerogel for nonsteroidal anti-inflammatory drugs controlled delivery systems using prilling and supercritical-assisted drying. Journal of Pharmaceutical Sciences. 2013;**102**(1):185-194. DOI: 10.1002/jps.23361

[74] Das S, Chaudhury A, Ng K-Y. Preparation and evaluation of zinc–pectin–chitosan composite particles for drug delivery to the colon: Role of chitosan in modifying in vitro and in vivo drug release. International Journal of Pharmaceutics. 2011;**406**(1-2):11-20. DOI: http://dx.doi.org/10.1016/j.ijpharm.2010.12.015

[75] Moneghini M, Bellich B, Baxa P, Princivalle F. Microwave generated solid dispersions containing Ibuprofen. International Journal of Pharmaceutics. 2008;**361**(1-2):125-130. DOI: http://dx.doi.org/10.1016/j.ijpharm.2008.05.026

[76] Jamuna-Thevi K, Zakaria FA, Othman R, Muhamad S. Development of macroporous calcium phosphate scaffold processed via microwave rapid drying. Materials Science and Engineering: C. 2009;**29**(5):1732-1740. DOI: 10.1016/j.msec.2009.01.022

[77] Gainotti A, Losi E, Colombo P, Santi P, Sonvico F, Baroni D, et al. The effect of residual water on antacid properties of sucralfate gel dried by microwaves. AAPS PharmSciTech. 2006;**7**(1):E58-E63.

[78] Bergese P, Colombo I, Gervasoni D, Depero LE. Microwave generated nanocomposites for making insoluble drugs soluble. Materials Science and Engineering: C. 2003;**23**(6-8):791-795. DOI: http://dx.doi.org/10.1016/j.msec.2003.09.137

[79] Nurjaya S, Wong TW. Effects of microwave on drug release properties of matrices of pectin. Carbohydrate Polymers. 2005;**62**(3):245-257.

[80] Wong TW, Chan LW, Kho SB, Heng PWS. Aging and microwave effects on alginate/chitosan matrices. Journal of Controlled Release. 2005;**104**(3):461-475. DOI: 10.1016/j.jconrel.2005.03.003

[81] Acierno D, Barba AA, d'Amore M, Pinto IM, Fiumara V. Microwaves in soil remediation from VOCs. 2. Buildup of a dedicated device. AIChE Journal. 2004;**50**(3):722-732.

[82] Wathey B, Tierney J, Lidström P, Westman J. The impact of microwave-assisted organic chemistry on drug discovery. Drug Discovery Today. 2002;**7**(6):373-380.

[83] Venkatesh M, Raghavan G. An overview of microwave processing and dielectric properties of agri-food materials. Biosystems Engineering. 2004;**88**(1):1-18.

[84] Içier F, Baysal T. Dielectrical properties of food materials—1: Factors affecting and industrial uses. Critical Reviews in Food Science and Nutrition. 2004;**44**(6):465-71.

[85] Auriemma G, Del Gaudio P, Barba AA, d'Amore M, Aquino RP. A combined technique based on prilling and microwave assisted treatments for the production of ketoprofen controlled release dosage forms. International Journal of Pharmaceutics. 2011;**415**(1-2):196-205.

[86] Araszkiewicz M, Koziola A, Lupinskaa A, Lupinskia M. Temperature distribution in a single sphere dried with microwaves and hot air. Drying Technology. 2006;**24**:1381-1386.

[87] Cirri M, Maestrelli F, Mennini N, Mura P. Physical-chemical characterization of binary and ternary systems of ketoprofen with cyclodextrins and phospholipids. Journal of Pharmaceutical and Biomedical Analysis. 2009;**50**(5):683-689. DOI: 10.1016/j.jpba.2008.11.003

[88] Vrečer F, Vrbinc M, Meden A. Characterization of piroxicam crystal modifications. International Journal of Pharmaceutics. 2003;**256**(1-2):3-15. http://dx.doi.org/10.1016/S0378-5173(03)00057-7

[89] García-González CA, Alnaief M, Smirnova I. Polysaccharide-based aerogels: Promising biodegradable carriers for drug delivery systems. Carbohydrate Polymers. 2011;**86**(4):1425-1438. DOI: http://dx.doi.org/10.1016/j.carbpol.2011.06.066

[90] Fricke J, Emmerling A. Aerogels—recent progress in production techniques and novel applications. Journal of Sol-Gel Science and Technology. 1998;**13**(1):299-303. DOI: 10.1023/a:1008663908431

[91] Larsen C, Østergaard J, Larsen SW, Jensen H, Jacobsen S, Lindegaard C, et al. Intra-articular depot formulation principles: Role in the management of postoperative pain and arthritic disorders. Journal of Pharmaceutical Sciences. 2008;**97**(11):4622-4654. DOI: 10.1002/jps.21346

[92] Hyllested M, Jones S, Pedersen JL, Kehlet H. Comparative effect of paracetamol, NSAIDs or their combination in postoperative pain management: A qualitative review. British Journal of Anaesthesia. 2002;**88**(2):199-214. DOI: 10.1093/bja/88.2.199

[93] Cooper S, Reynolds D, Reynolds B, Hersh E. Analgesic efficacy and safety of (R)-ketoprofen in postoperative dental pain. Journal of Clinical Pharmacology. 1998;**38**(2 Suppl):11S-18S.

[94] Holdgate A, Pollock T. Nonsteroidal anti-inflammatory drugs (NSAIDS) versus opioids for acute renal colic. Cochrane Database of Systematic Reviews. 2004(1). DOI: 10.1002/14651858.CD004137.pub3.

[95] Papadoukakis S, Stolzenburg J-U, Truss MC. Treatment strategies of ureteral stones. EAU-EBU Update Series. 2006;**4**(5):184-190. DOI: 10.1016/j.eeus.2006.07.004

[96] Reverchon E, De Marco I. Supercritical fluid extraction and fractionation of natural matter. Journal of Supercritical Fluids. 2006;**38**(2):146-166. DOI: 10.1016/j.supflu.2006.03.020

[97] Cardea S, Pisanti P, Reverchon E. Generation of chitosan nanoporous structures for tissue engineering applications using a supercritical fluid assisted process. Journal of Supercritical Fluids. 2010;**54**(3):290-295. DOI: 10.1016/j.supflu.2010.05.014

[98] Aquino RP, Auriemma G, d'Amore M, D'Ursi AM, Mencherini T, Del Gaudio P. Piroxicam loaded alginate beads obtained by prilling/microwave tandem technique: Morphology and drug release. Carbohydrate Polymers. 2012;**89**(3):740-748. DOI: http://dx.doi.org/10.1016/j.carbpol.2012.04.003

[99] Kocbek P, Baumgartner S, Kristl J. Preparation and evaluation of nanosuspensions for enhancing the dissolution of poorly soluble drugs. International Journal of Pharmaceutics. 2006;**312**(1-2):179-186.

Chapter 5

Nonsteroidal Anti-inflammatory Drugs: Integrated Approach to Physical Medicine and Rehabilitation

Rosa Grazia Bellomo, Simona Maria Carmignano,
Tommaso Palermo, Lucia Cosenza,
Andrea Saggini and Raoul Saggini

Additional information is available at the end of the chapter

http://dx.doi.org/10.5772/intechopen.69257

Abstract

Inflammation is an immediate response to damage; in acute phase, it is a form of defense for body and it aims to restitutio ad integrum, in the chronic form itself becomes disease. This mechanism determines inflammatory diseases that are a group of clinical disorders which are characterized by abnormal inflammatory responses such as osteoarthritis, in myalgic syndromes (like fibromyalgia or miofascial sindrome), in some forms of headache, in peripheral vascular disease, in many malignancies. In Physical and Rehabilitation Medicine, the use of analgesic drugs (including NSAIDs) is a crucial resource inside a complex bioprogressive rehabilitative project. A part of the classic use per os is characterized by a serious and systemic side effect and there is also a possibility to administer drugs through other routes. Antalgic and rehabilitative mesotherapy (ARM) is a minimally invasive technique consisting of subcutaneous injections of bioactive substances. Other alternatives are represented by iontophoresis, phonophoresis, phytotherapy, and topical application. The purpose of this chapter is to give an overview about the state of the art regarding the use of NSAIDs in physical medicine and rehabilitation.

Keywords: NSAIDs, antalgic and rehabilitative mesotherapy, iontophoresis, phonophoresis, phytotherapy

1. Inflammation

Inflammation is an immediate response to damage to tissues and cells by pathogens, noxious stimuli such as chemicals, or physical injury. Already in the short-term, there is an attempt at healing with white blood cells that arrive in the damaged area for repair process. Chronic inflammation, indeed, is a prolonged response that involves active inflammation, tissue destruction, and delays repair. Chronic and persistent inflammation is associated with many chronic human conditions and diseases, including allergy, atherosclerosis, cancer, arthritis, and autoimmune diseases. Acute inflammation is characterized by abrupt onset, followed by a rapid succession of events (hours or days) essentially vascular (hence angiophlogosis) responsible for the cardinal signs, culminating in the resolution or chronicity. Chronic inflammation has greater duration of the previous form (months or years), with oscillations of the gravity and phenomena of intensifcation during its evolution. It is also defined as istophlogosis, for the prevalence of tissue phenomena due to infiltration of mononuclear blood cells [1]. The cardinal symptoms of inflammation, described by the Roman physician Aulus Cornelius Celsus (30 before Christ - 38 Anno Domini), are: calor, rubor, tumor, dolor, who later Galen (130–200 AD) added functio laesa, indicating the functional impairment.

Inflammation process is a reaction triggered by innate immunity mechanisms, which evolved in a pattern that can vary based on etiologic agent, the headquarters of the damage and the intensity of the damage.

The mechanism underlying inflammation process is connected to the physiological state of homeostasis. Several studies suggest that inflammation operates as a much-sophisticated system than ever thought at the molecular level. The inflammation is mainly a local reaction, which generates a systemic response when it exceeds a certain threshold and molecules, synthesized and released into bloodstream in response to the damage, acting on distant organs that express receptors for them. As longer this response persists in the host will encounter the more damaging consequences [2]. Increased vascular permeability, that is a feature of acute inflammation, leading to the leakage of a protein-rich fluid (exudate) in the interstitium, to this, follows a variation of interstitial pressure (increases) and intravascular pressure (decreases). The presence of exudate and the hydrostatic pressure difference, draws fluid in the interstitial tissue with net result of edema. The first cellular step is represented by inflammatory stimuli that are first recognized by the host cells through specific transmembrane receptors, called pattern recognition receptors (PRRs), which are expressed by cells of both innate and adaptive immune systems. PRRs are responsible for sensing the presence of infecting microorganisms as well as the incidence of any cellular injuries. Disintegration of the tissue cells affected (with relative release of intracellular substances) determines the mobilization, through the blood, of the immune cells that reach the site of the lesion to begin a defence and repair process (activities mediated by substances released by these same cells) [3].

Once activated the inflammatory response, we see the release of chemical mediators that quickly induce alterations in the microcirculation, i.e., the vessels interposed between the

http://dx.doi.org/10.5772/intechopen.69257

small arteries and small veins, arterioles, capillaries and venules. Thus, it began the vascular phase of inflammation, characterized by vasodilation and increased permeability.

The cells of the host's immunocompetent system also (among which should be mentioned macrophages, polymorphonuclear granulocytes, the mast cells, fibroblasts and platelets) contribute to the process. Subsequently, mediators such as bradicin, histamine, serotonin (5-HT, 5-HydroxyTriptamine), prostaglandins (prostaglandins (PGs), cytokines (including Interleukin (IL) and tumor necrosis factor (TNF) and some nerve growth factors Fabric, including nerve growth factor (NGF), neurotrophic factor derived from glial cell line (GDNF) and the neurotrophic factor derived from the brain (BDNF), are released [4]. Furthermore, it must consider the role of cyclooxygenase 2 (Cox-2, cycle-oxygenase-2), enzymes that, by acting inside of fibroblasts, favour the production of PGs, which have a great importance in causing inflammation and the ache. To complete the process of the liberated substances and widespread during the inflammatory process, among these must be counted calcitonin gene-related peptide (CGRP), which activates the nociceptors, and Nitric oxide (NO), gas with great ability to spread among tissues and responsible for the neurotoxic effects. A neurochemical response from the same nerve cells is involved in pain perception (neurogenic inflammation). The damaged cells release a large amount of chemicals, including, in particular, some ions (mainly hydrogen ions, H+, responsible for local acidosis) and adenosine triphosphate (ATP) [5, 6]. (**Figure 1**)

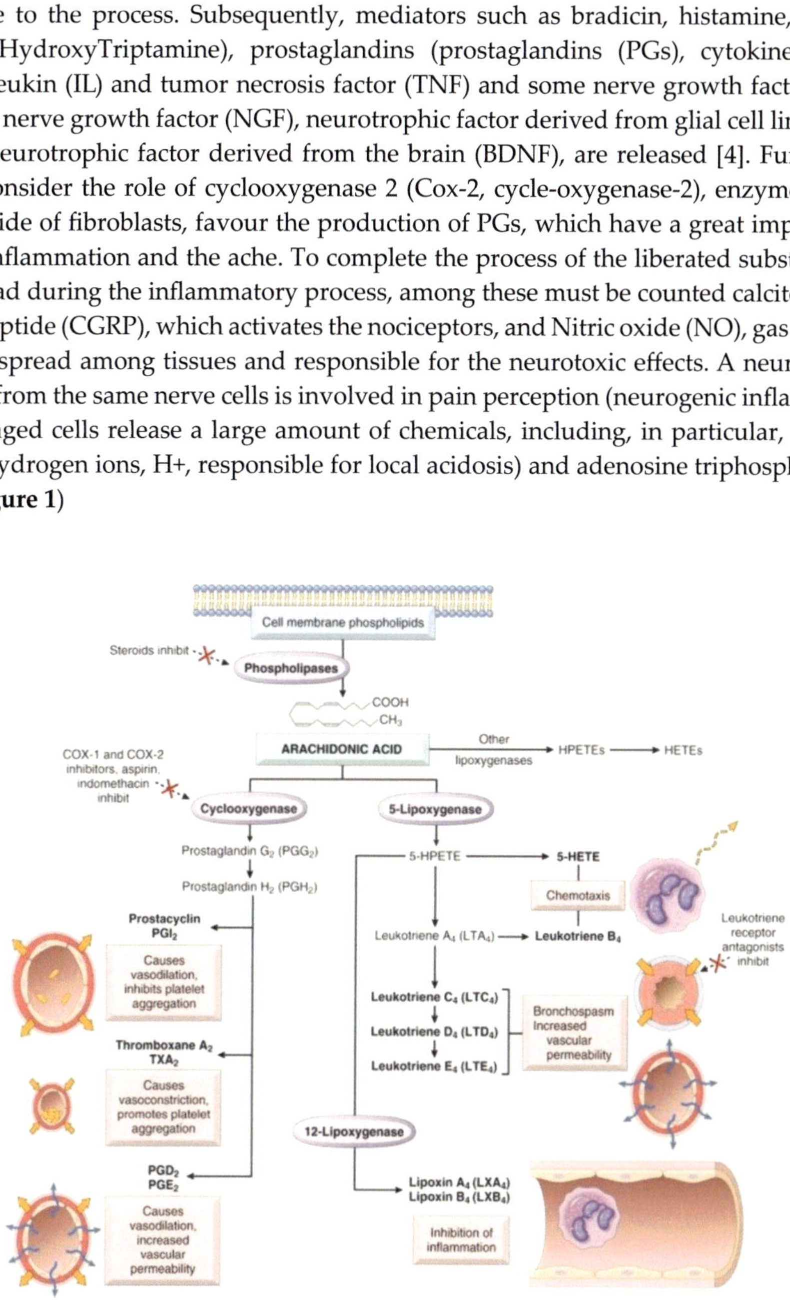

Figure 1. Inflammatory process.

All these substances have an active role in the onset of pain, a phenomenon closely related to inflammation [7]. Since the sensory nerve endings possess a variety of receptors designed to bind with the inflammatory mediators, some of the freed molecules such as adenosine triphosphate and hydrogen ions, act on nociceptors, activating them directly and causing an immediate depolarization, starting a painful stimulus. Other substances, instead, act on other receptors that are not able to start the painful stimulus but which are capable of sensitizing nociceptors, or to lower the activation threshold. While the first category of brokers, the depolarizing substances, causes pain, the second category, that of sensitizing substances, causes hyperalgesia. Among the substances that sensitize the receptors necessary to signal, there is the serotonin (5-HT), which is commonly released from platelets and mast cells in damaged tissue and inflamed. It acts by activating two receptor subtypes (5-HT2 and 5-HT3 receptor), whose action is synergistic with that of the receptors for bradykinin and for PGs. An inflammatory process of a somatic structure is manifested in particular with pain of varying intensity in relation to the release of active chemical mediators on algo-sensitive endings. Spinal reflexes of defence, through an increase in skeletal muscle tension, and hyperactivity of the sympathetic, contribute to the alteration of the microenvironment and the maintenance of the effects on nociceptors. The ultimate step in the elimination of traumatic agents and necrotic cells is their degradation within neutrophils and macrophages, which occur most efficiently after activation of the phagocytes. An efficacy system of host defence minimizes the damage and finally it controls the end of process. In fact, inflammation declines simply because the mediators of inflammation have short half-lives, but also because stop signals are released, they block the process [8].

In this way, in fact, the switch of arachidonic acid's metabolism acts toward the production of anti-inflammatory lipoxins, the release of transforming growth factor-β (TGF-β), an anti-inflammatory cytokine, from macrophages and other cells; and the cholinergic discharge that inhibit the production of TNF in macrophages [9].

The acute inflammation turns into a chronic one, when the process of resolution fails. Pathological states characterized by chronic inflammation are still under investigation, because in the West there are a great number of patients with these conditions, and also because the mechanisms that underlie chronic inflammation are not yet well understood. Chronic diseases, often, are not triggered by infections or pathogens and this make the understanding of their pathological processes much more complicated [10]. Chronic phlogosis is the cause of these conditions and it is not derived by xenobiotics, but it is generated by inflammatory cells that act against the host itself. This mechanism determines inflammatory diseases that are a group of clinical disorders which are characterized by abnormal inflammatory responses such as osteoarthritis, in myalgic syndromes (like fibromyalgia), in some forms of headache, in peripheral vascular disease, and in many malignancies [11].

2. From pathophysiology to pharmacology

The study of inflammatory pathophysiology was crucial stimulus to the search for substances pharmaceutically active on related symptoms. NSAIDs are mainly anti-inflammatory, but also analgesic and antipyretic drugs. They are typically used in the treatment of pain, to reduce stiffness, and to enhance function in patients with musculoskeletal disorders, osteoarthritis, rheumatoid arthritis, and other forms of arthritis. Furthermore, NSAIDs are also used for the treatment of acute pain including headache, dysmenorrhea, and postoperative pain [12, 13].

Acetylsalicylic acid (ASA), better known as aspirin, is the prototypical NSAID. ASA traces its origins back to willow bark, a natural source of the chemical salicylate. All NSAIDs interrupt the production of inflammatory and pain-related hormones called prostaglandins. The isolation of salicylic acid in the nineteenth century from willow and poplar barks led to its widespread use as an antipyretic, analgesic and anti-inflammatory agent. Since then, many nonsteroidal compounds with anti-inflammatory properties have been discovered. Since ASA's introduction in 1897, more than two dozen chemically-related drugs have been developed. The group is generally restricted only to those substances that act by inhibiting components of the enzyme system in the metabolism of arachidonic acid and formation of eicosanoids. Key pharmaceutical class is that of NSAIDs, which act on the metabolism of arachidonic acid, reducing the production of prostaglandins that intervene on the vascular phase of inflammation and sensitize nociceptors by lowering the activation threshold by algogenic substances. Prostaglandins' synthesis part from phospholipids commonly contained in the membrane structure of all cells, which, by enzymatic action effect of phosphorylase, is transformed into arachidonic acid: this molecule acting on the cyclooxygenases 1 and 2 (Cox-1 and Cox -2), which are responsible for the synthesis of PGs. PGs, in turn, act on the prostaglandin receptors (EP) and this activation is derived from a particular sensitization of nociceptors, able to produce hyperalgesia. Many common drugs used for joint pain, rheumatism, but also fever, act by inhibiting the COX-1 or COX-2, or both, and reducing, among other things, pain and hyperalgesia. The COX binds the NSAIDs on an arginine residue (ARG120) and from here the inhibitory part of the drug clutters the active site of "enzyme; in fact the" enzyme is bifunctional and has two active sites, one that transforms the "acid in PGG2 and another that turns this" last in PGH2, but NSAIDs inhibit the first of the two sites. It is a reversible competitive inhibition, with the exception of aspirin, which binds instead to Serina 530 with an irreversible bond. Its effect, therefore, lasts even after the deletion of the medication from body, as long as it is not synthesized new enzyme. The various NSAIDs, presently, can be divided on the basis of their selectivity to COX.

The COX-1 is a constitutive enzyme expressed in most cells, responsible for the physiological production of prostanoids, ubiquitous mediators that, through the interaction of specific membrane receptors coupled with G proteins, are involved in intercellular communication and in the modulation of several homeostatic functions (gastric, platelets, kidney).

COX-2 is inducible isoform of the enzyme as a result of pro-inflammatory stimuli, mainly responsible for the production of prostanoid mediators of inflammation and in pain transmission. However, in the CNS, kidney, prostate, testes, and vessels are COX-2 of constitutive type. Inhibition of COX-2 by NSAIDs, should be responsible for the therapeutic effects, whereas inhibition of COX-1 would result in adverse reactions to these drugs. The COXIB are selective inhibitors of COX-2.

NSAIDs are classified as in **Figure 2**.

It was estimated that about 100 million people worldwide use NSAIDs and therefore are the most widely used drugs ever, especially in the treatment of postoperative pain and pain related to musculoskeletal disorders (Berde and Sundel) such as rheumatoid arthritis or osteoarthritis [14].

Diclofenac has anti-inflammatory analgesic and antipyretic effect, and its power is greater than other NSAIDs. It is indicated for chronic inflammatory diseases such as rheumatoid arthritis and osteoarthritis at a dose of 100–200 mg/day. It is also used as analgesic in the case of musculoskeletal injuries, tendinitis, postoperative pain, and dysmenorrhea (50 mg). It is rapidly absorbed after oral administration and has a short half-life of 1–2 hours. A new salt of diclofenac, diclofenac epolamine, is highly effective as both an anti-inflammatory and an analgesic agent for its favourable permeation characteristics. Furthermore, recently, it is put commercially a new formulation of diclofenac injectable, diclofenac sodium together with cyclodextrins, which improves the solubility of diclofenac. It is a new pharmaceutical form in 1 ml volume which offers not only the unique advantage of the subcutaneous administration (besides the "classical" intra-muscular injection) but also the use of the lowest dosage.

Ketorolac (LIXIDOL, Toradol): It is a potent analgesic and a moderate anti-inflammatory. Unlike opioid analgesics, it does not give tolerance, dependence, and respiratory depression. It uses intramuscular (30–90 mg) for the treatment of post-operative pain as an alternative to opioids.

It acts in the reduction of post-surgical pain (arthroplasty, disc herniations, femoral fractures with reduction). It is also used in the most difcult forms of dysmenorrhea, or for the treatment of renal colic sporadic and chronic.

Salicylates • Acetylsalicylic acid (aspirin) • Amoxiprin • Benorylate/Benorilate • Choline magnesium salicylate • Diflunisal • Ethenzamide • Faislamine • Methyl salicylate • Magnesium salicylate • Salicyl salicylate • Salicylamide	Arylalkanoic acids • Diclofenac • Aceclofenac • Acemethacin • Alclofenac • Bromfenac • Etodolac • Indomethacin • Nabumetone • Oxametacin • Proglumetacin • Sulindac • Tolmetin	2-Arylpropionic acids (profens) • Ibuprofen • Alminoprofen • Carprofen • Dexibuprofen • Dexketoprofen • Fenbufen • Fenoprofen • Flunoxaprofen • Flurbiprofen • Indoprofen • Ketorolac • Loxoprofen • Naproxen • Oxaprozin • Pirprofen • Suprofen • Tiaprofenic acid	N-Arylanthranilic acids (fenamic acids) • Mefenamic acid • Flufenamic acid • Meclofenamic acid • Tolfenamic acid
Pyrazolidine derivatives • Phenylbutazone • Ampyrone • Azapropazone • Clofezone • Kebuzone • Metamizole • Mofebutazone • Oxyphenbutazone • Phenazone • Sulfinpyrazone	Oxicams • Piroxicam • Droxicam • Lornoxicam • Meloxicam • Tenoxicam	[COX]-2 inhibitors • Celecoxib (FDA alert) • Etoricoxib (FDA withdrawn) • Lumiracoxib TGA cancelled registration • Parecoxib FDA withdrawn • Rofecoxib (withdrawn from market) • Valdecoxib (withdrawn from market)	

Figure 2. Classification of NSAIDs.

Treatment with ketorolac should not exceed 5 days to the possibility of serious complications gastric, haemorrhagic, and renal.

Ibuprofen (Brufen, MOMENT) is used as anti-inflammatory for rheumatoid arthritis, osteoarthritis, periarthritis, low back pain, sciatica at a dose of 2400 mg/day. At lower doses, it is devoid of anti-inflammatory activity and is used as an analgesic in various forms including painful headache and dysmenorrhoea (400 mg every 4–6 hours).

It has a short half-life of 1–2 hours; it is highly bound to plasma proteins and it does not interact with anticoagulants.

Naproxen (ALEVE, FLOGINAX, Naprosyn, Naprosyn GEL, NAPRIUS, MOMENDOL, SYNFLEX). It has the same pharmacological profile and the same indications of ibuprofen. It is a well-tolerated drug. It has long half-life of 12–15 hours. The half-life is approximately doubled in elderly patients thus making it necessary dosage changes.

Ketoprofen (Fastum, Orudis): It inhibits both COX and LPX. This property does not make it superior than others NSAIDS. The efficacy of ketoprofen in the treatment of rheumatoid arthritis and osteoarthritis is similar to that of aspirin and other NSAIDs. It has a very short half-life of 1–2 hours; it is highly bound to plasma proteins, but does not modify the activity of warfarin and digoxin. Probenecid increases the plasma levels and prolongs the half-life [15].

The World Health Organization (WHO) in 1996 proposed a scale for pain assessment in the first instance oncological and later adopted as a guideline for the pharmacological treatment of musculoskeletal pain. This scale consists of three levels:

- Pain Mild (assessment of pain according to visual analogue scale—VAS from 1 to 4): it is suggested treatment with NSAIDs or acetaminophen ± adjuvants.
- Pain Mild to moderate (VAS 5-6): it is suggested treatment with weak opioids or NSAIDs ± paracetamol ± adjuvants.
- Pain Severe or moderate to severe (VAS 7-10): it is suggested treatment with strong opioids ± NSAIDs or acetaminophen ± adjuvants [16] (**Figure 3**).

The chronic use of NSAIDs cause: coagulopathies (reduced platelet aggregation, increased bleeding time), gastrointestinal toxicity (gastritis and dyspepsia, ulcers, vomiting blood, diarrhoea), hepatotoxicity (increased transaminases, cholestatic hepatitis, acute hepatic necrosis), haematological effects (leukopenia, agranulocytosis, aplastic anemia), kidney effects (salt and water retention, azotemia, oliguria, interstitial nephritis, papillary necrosis, acute), respiratory effects (bronchospasm), allergy, dermatitis, headache.

NSAIDs interactions with other drugs: reduce the efficacy of beta-blockers, ACE-inhibitors and diuretics; increase the effect of sulfonylureas and toxicity of aminoglycosides and cyclosporine. The COXIB, long-term, increases the risk of serious cardiovascular events and thrombosis, myocardial infarction, stroke; also, such as NSAIDs, increase the risk of serious gastrointestinal adverse effects (bleeding, ulceration and perforation), even in the absence of warning symptoms [17].

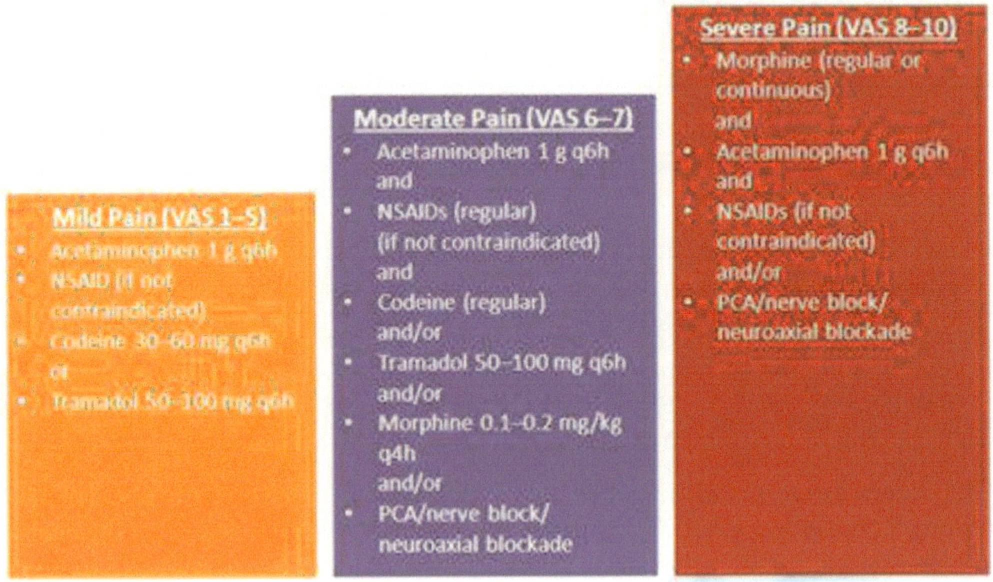

Figure 3. The World Health Organization (WHO) scale for pain assessment in the first instance oncological and later adopted as a guideline for the pharmacological treatment.

To minimize or abolish the adverse effects of the oral administration of these drugs, there are several techniques used in physical and rehabilitation medicine, such as mesotherapy, iontophoresis, phonophoresis, and last but not least, phytotherapy which uses natural substances with anti-inflammatory properties.

3. Antalgic and rehabilitative mesotherapy

Mesotherapy is based on the principle that intradermal therapy produces a "micro deposit" of the drug in the dermis which is then slowly released into the surrounding tissues. Nowadays, mesotherapy should be considered an increasingly important aspect of Interventional Physical and Rehabilitation Medicine (IPRM).

Mesotherapy consists of a series of "microinjections" of drug/active substance into the dermis using short needles where the needle is positioned at an appropriate angle depending on the thickness of the skin. A French physician, Michel Pistor, reporting encouraging results with small drugs administered intradermically to patients with a variety of clinical condition. He defines mesotherapy as a novel analgesic therapy for a variety of rheumatologic disorders [18, 19]. The term mesotherapy derives from Greek (Mesos = "Medium" and Therapeia = "care"), and refers to the mesoderm germ layer from which are differentiated tissues and structures such as bone, cartilage, muscle and connective tissue. It makes superficial injections directly on the area above the structure affected by the disease, using a 27–33 gauge needle; typically administered are 0.10–0.20 ml of medication and injection points at 2–3 cm distance.

http://dx.doi.org/10.5772/intechopen.69257

Although the fundamental principles upon which mesotherapy are those expressed by Michel Pistor, mesotherapy concept evolved in recent years: from the concept of needle insertion in the point of greatest pain (such as trigger points) to injection of analgesic agents such as lidocaine or bicarbonate, [20, 21] arriving at the concept of mesotherapy as aspect of Interventional Physical and Rehabilitation Medicine (IPRM). The Interventional Physical and Rehabilitation Medicine (IPRM) is the possibility by physiatrist to insert in the individual rehabilitation project, with the most appropriate timing, an interventional procedure to support the conservative applied methods. In addition, mesotherapy is a procedure in which not only is it possible to introduce a specific drug, but it represents the possibility to choose whether to treat the point of maximum pain, the area of referred pain or functional damaged district. Depending on the needle technique used, it is possible to reach different tissues and different depths. The use of more deep techniques, associated with the administration of the drug, can interrupt the inflammatory cascade and it generates, as a result of the mechanical action of the needle, tissue repair processes with reduction of local fibrosis.

There are various techniques of mesotherapy that are different depending on the used needle length and gauge, the injected substance, the depth of penetration:

Intraepidermic (IED) in which the injection is carried out at the level of the epidermis-dermis junction at 1–2 mm depth with the needle parallel to the skin and the bevel of the needle faces upwards.

Nappagein in which is recommended a deeper injection at 2–4 mm with an angle of 30–60 degrees. Usually two to four injections are carried out with a space of 3–4 mm between each point of injection.

Point-by-point (PPP) with a deep injections at 4 mm at most.

Mesoperfusion in which injections should be involved at 4–13 mm over 30–90 minutes.

The perfect drug for mesotherapy is the one whose technical data sheet covering three routes for parenteral administration. If a certain drug or association exists both intramuscular and intravenous version, the first is preferred, because the tissues of mesotherapy—epidermis, dermis and subcutaneous—have greater histochemical affinity with muscle rather than blood.

The most commonly used in mesotherapy drugs are NSAIDs (diclofenac, ketoprofen, aspirin, ketorolac, piroxicam), muscle relaxants (thiocolchicoside, pridinolo mesylate), vasoactive drugs (mesoglycan), calcium chelators (EDTA) and local anesthetics (lidocaine, procaine). Diclofenac sodium together with ciclodextrins is a solution for injection can be administered intramuscularly or subcutaneously as mesotheraphy. It can be used in different doses: in case of mild or moderate pain, it is sufficient to use the lowest dose (25 mg). A dose of 50–75 mg may be required in case of severe pain. Exceptionally and in severe cases, it can be administered a second dose of 75 mg after six hours. The maximum daily dose (24 hours) must not exceed 150 mg.

They should never be injected mesotherapy turbid drugs or frankly precipitating, since the crystals also of small size can obstruct thin blood capillaries and determine thrombosis and tissue necrosis. To avoid the reaction of acid-basic cocktail with opposite pH products, you can load the syringe with the defined quantity of saline at the beginning of the preparation. Each cocktail drug must be diluted in physiological solution in the volumetric ratio of 1:10 or 0.5 ml:5 ml. In mesotherapy it is prohibited inject oily and alcoholic solutions for the high risk of necrosis. Corticosteroids are contraindicated both individually and in cocktails because it can cause skin atrophy. In the case of extra-articular injections it is a side effect with estimated frequency from Brinks et al. [22] of around 1%, but with possible serious aesthetic impact, which in intradermal injections is likely much higher [23].

The risk of allergic reactions preclude the intradermal administration of a muscle relaxant plus a nonsteroidal anti-inflammatory agent in the same syringe as it is not possible to determinate which drug has caused the allergy.

Protocols for mesotherapy allow to make one or more cycles depending on the symptoms, the severity of the disease and the patient's response. In chronic painful conditions there are three distinct phases: attack (sevently weekly treatments are administrated), control (four fortnightly treatments are given to confirm results and prevent short-term recurrences) and maintenance phase (monthly or seasonal treatment). In resistant pain, twice weekly therapy is recommended in the "attack phase" depending on the analgesic effect obtained. There are several advantages of mesotherapy: the process of introducing needles into the skin stimulates a reflex action thereby increasing endorphin levels, which blocks the painful sensation; the rapidity of action, related to the short time required to reach the site of action, as well as a prolonged local effect and a reduction of side effects.

The use of mesotherapy in Italy was approved by the Italian Society of Mesotherapy (SIM) in 1975, following a number of multi-center studies have confirmed the effectiveness of this method in the control of joint pain (hip/knee osteoarthritis/Hand, neck pain, back pain, tendonitis) (**Figure 4**).

In addition to the analgesic and anti-inflammatory effect, these studies have demonstrated the safety of administration and reduction of side effects compared to oral via.

The combined use of mesotherapy with physical therapy achieves a synergistic effect in muscle injuries of athletes, control of neuropathic pain, inflammatory tendonitis, degenerative and/or calcified. The indication more appropriately, according to these studies, is treatment of musculoskeletal and osteo-articular pain. Open studies conducted with mesotheraphy approach in musculoskeletal pain such us arthritis, neck pain, lower back pain, and tendinopathy show a reduction of pain at least 50% compared to pre-treatment [24–39].

Furthermore, literature reported that a great number of patients treated with mesotherapy for musculoskeletal pain disorders had rapid pain relief, generally when the patient responds within the first three sessions of therapy [40].

Costantino et al., started a study with the aim to compare mesotherapic versus conventional systemic administration of nonsteroidal anti-inflammatory drugs (NSAIDs) and corticosteroids in patients with acute low back pain. They showed that the administration of NSAIDs and corticosteroids via mesotherapy can provide the same therapeutic benefit as that induced by conventional (oral and intramuscular) drug administration. The major aspect is the comparable effectiveness of mesotherapy and conventional systemic therapy, despite the lower

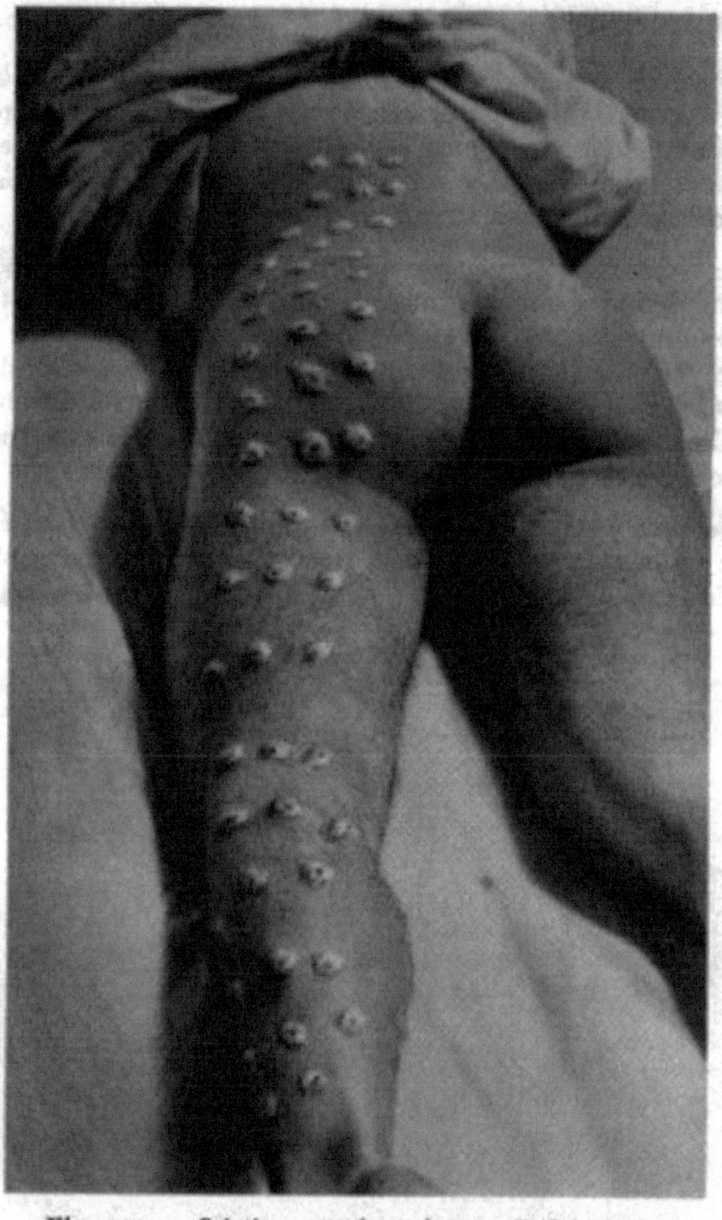

Fig. 113. — *Sciatique gauche. 2 à 3 cc. d'Algipan sont répartis tout le long du trajet sciatique douloureux.*

Figure 4. Mesotherapy in 1975, low back pain and sciatica.

amount of drugs administered to patients undergoing mesotherapy (41.67% ketoprofen and 50% methylprednisolone). Author concluded that subcutaneous drug administration results in a very slow drug absorption such as intramuscular and oral and that it could be assumed that anti-inflammatory substances, dispensed with mesotherapy, reach a high drug concentration into the subcutaneous tissue and it acts locally close to the inflammatory cells, sensitive fibers and vascular mediators that generate inflammation and pain [41].

Even in the case of carpal tunnel syndrome, diagnosed by clinical examination and neurophysiological investigation, it used a mixture containing lidocaine 10 mg, ketoprofen lysine-acetylsalycilate 80 mg, xantinol nicotinato 100 mg, cyanocobalamin 1000 mcg more injectable water, injected above the transverse carpal ligament, at the base of the thenar and hypothenar eminence. It has noticed already after 24 hours, a significant reduction in pain and paresthesias, which lasted up to 12 months in over 50% of the sample.

The mesotherapy with NSAIDs is applicable to several pathological conditions, as demonstrated by several studies, starting from pes anserine bursitis, treated by Saggini et al. (**Figure 5**) with nine sessions of mesotherapy with diclofenac sodium (25 mg/1 ml; Akis, IBSA, Switzerland), 1 ml per session, three times a week. These patients' outcome was assessed by visual analogue scale (VAS), along with the ability to perform activities of daily life, the ability to participate in sports, level of pain, symptoms, and quality of life. These measurements were performed before and after the treatment period and at 30 and 90 days of follow up. It was thus obtained with a significant reduction in pain after the treatment period; further

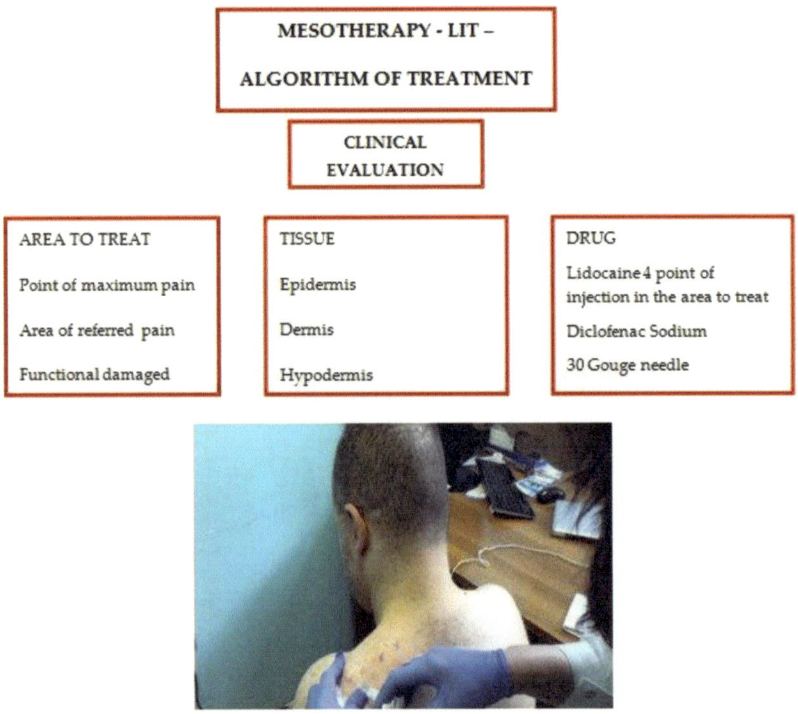

Figure 5. Algorithm treatment of antalgic and rehabilitative mesotherapy. Center of Physical and Rehabilitation Medicine, "Gabriele d'Annunzio" University, Chieti- Chief R. Saggini md.

ultrasound investigations showed a hypoechoic area reduction related to pes anserine bursitis only in the group receiving mesotherapy and not in the control group, treated, however, with oral therapy [42].

The mesotherapy is therefore an innovative technique specific of Interventional Physical and Rehabilitation Medicine (IPRM). It enables operation of painful conditions also chronic, inflammatory, degenerative, and traumatic diseases. This type of therapy, which can be defined "ecological," fits perfectly into the global bioprogressive approach, where to work on the bone-myofascial system, this must be put in the control condition and reduction of pain, to optimize dynamics of the body and thus increase performance.

4. Iontophoresis

The method of iontophoresis has been described by Pivati in 1747. In the eighteenth century, two illustrious scientists Galvani and Volta, joined together the principle by which electrons' movement generate electricity and that according to which electricity moves ions [43] (**Figure 6**). In the 1870s, the German Hermann Munk (1839–1912) extensively investigated the current mediated transport of substances, such as strychnine, through porous membranes. He then thought about transmitting drugs through intact human skin as the skin is some kind of a porous membrane as well. The strychnine experiments were repeated by the French physician

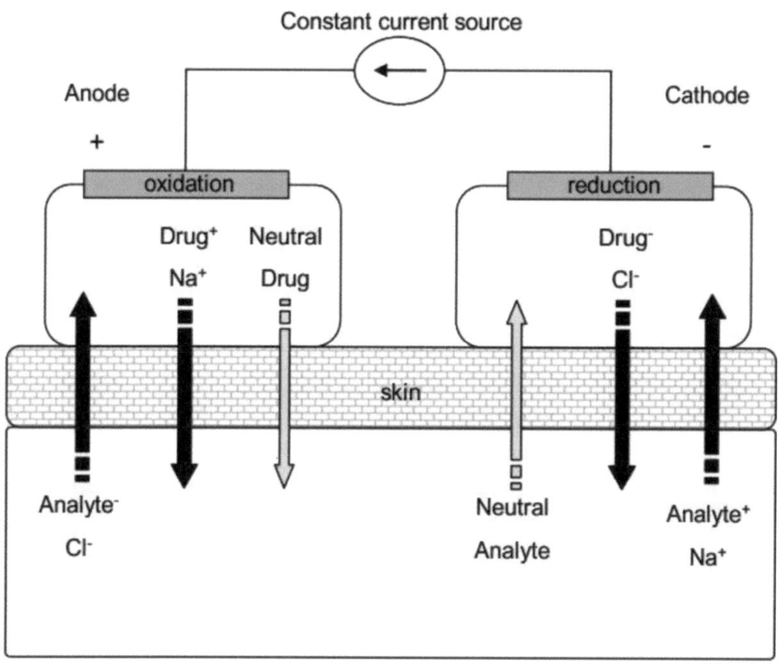

Figure 6. Molecular transport during iontophoresis.

Stéphane Leduc (1853–1939), showing that strychnine sulfate is transported from the positive to the negative pole of the electric circuit.

This phenomenon was intensively studied by Fritz Frankenhäuser (born 1868) who invented the term "Iontophorese" earlier than 1908 [44].

Iontophoresis is applied in physical medicine to treat musculoskeletal disorders such as osteoarthritis, bursitis, and tendinopathy by transdermal drug administration. It is a procedure that uses the application of a constant voltage electricity to convey through the skin charged and highly polar molecules. Iontophoretic transport can occur by electrorepulsion or electromigration, but considering the properties of the skin, drug can be transported by electro-osmosis [45].

The migration of the therapeutic agent also depends on its charge: cationic or neutral substances are conveyed toward the anode, anionic substances are conveyed toward the cathode. Applying a low voltage current, following the principle dell'elettro repulsion, the ions are repelled through the skin. Since the skin is negatively charged under physiological conditions, the electroosmotic flow is then from anode to cathode [46].

Restrictions about iontophoretic system, include law limits on the amount of current that can be used in humans (nowadays set to 0.5 mA/cmq) and the irreversible harm that such currents could do to the skin's barrier properties. Furthermore, iontophoresis has not managed to significantly improve the transdermal vehiculation of molecules >7000 Dalton [47].

The limit of mulecular size can be overcome with electroporation, i.e., the application of high voltage pulses to induce modifcations of skin.

Electroporation uses high voltages (≥100 V) for short treatment periods (milliseconds), which increase the skin permeability, probably for the generation of transient pores during electroporation. The result of electroporation is not always better than iontophoresis, but appears lasts longer. It depends on the energy of the electrical field [48]. (**Figure 7**)

Many factors influence the outcome of the transdermal delivery of drugs: physicochemical properties of the substance (charge, concentration, size of molecules), formulation (pH, viscosity, presence of other ions), biological variation (age, sex, site of application, vascularization), body temperature, types of electrodes and current used, duration of the session. (**Table 1**)

The main advantage of the transdermal administration of drugs, is the increased bioavailability of the active principle in absence of hepatic first-pass metabolism [49]. This hypothesis was tested for numerous NSAIDs in both in vitro and in vivo studies [50, 51]. In vitro, it has been demonstrated that piroxicam gel solution diffusion through the skin is 100–1000 fold higher applying iontophoresis for 6 hours, compared to the passive diffusion [52].

Also in vivo on man, it has been demonstrated this advantage of iontophoresis and it has been noticed a concentration of piroxicam in the stratum corneum significantly higher compared to the passive diffusion [53]. In another study in vitro, ketorolac has been convey through rat skin applying a current density from 0.11 to 0.15 mA/cmq with 10–100 fold increase than its passive vehiculation [54]. (**Figure 8**)

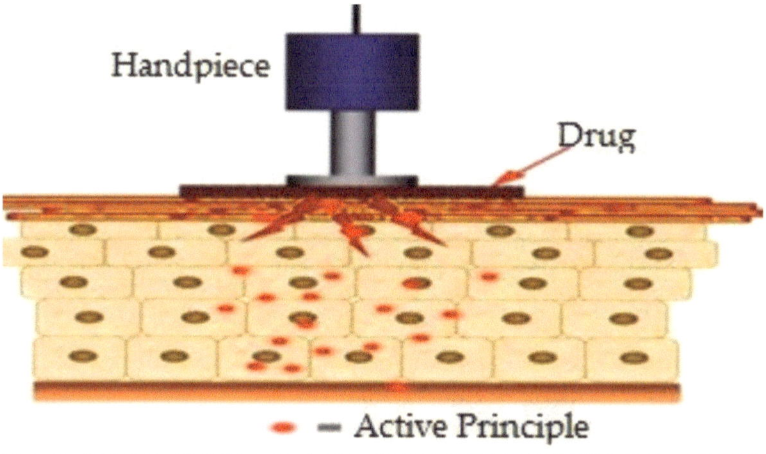

Figure 7. Electroporation.

Drug	Polarity
Lysine acetylsalicylate	Negative
Diclofenac sodium	Negative
Indomethacin	Negative
Piroxicam	Negative
Ketoprofen	Negative
Benzydamine hydrochloride	Bipolar
Methyl nicotinate	Positive
Phenylbutazone	Positive
Glycol salicylate	Positive

Table 1. Polarity of NSAIDs.

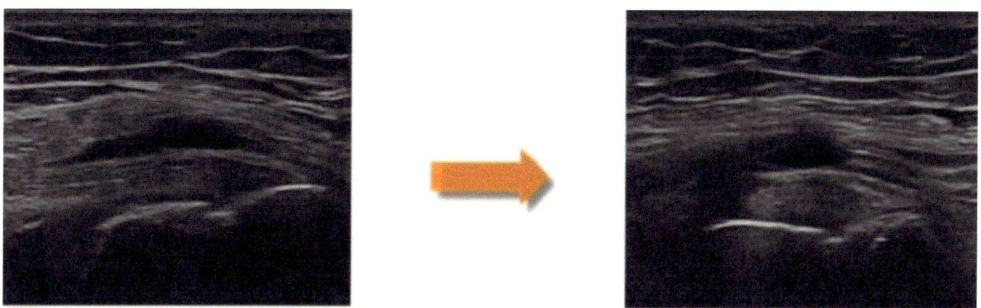

Figure 8. Ultrasonography: reduction of a hypoechoic area (pes anserine)—pre (T0) and after (T1) the treatment period: 30 days of transdermal diclofenac sodium 25 mg/ml with electroporation(Isofor Compact) for three times a week for three weeks with sessions lasting 20 minutes each. Center of Physical and Rehabilitation Medicine, "Gabriele d'Annunzio" University, Chieti- Chief R.Saggini MD.

A series of studies reported anti-inflammatory effects of iontophoresis and electroporation in many common inflammatory conditions of the musculoskeletal system. All of the clinical investigations demonstrated at least positive clinical outcome [55–58].

One of the first studies on the transdermal drug delivery goes back to 1996 by Saggini et al. in the treatment of rheumatic pain with ketorolac compared with placebo. Seven days after the end of therapy, patients who received ketorolac have experienced a further reduction in pain (highly significant compared to pre-treatment values; $P < 0.005$). The best results were observed in patients who had severe or very strong pain at the beginning of treatment. The intensity of pain in patients who received placebo, returned to pre-treatment values [59].

Baskurt et al. conducted a study comparing the effectiveness of transcutaneous delivery of naproxen via iontophoresis versus phonophoresis. The results suggest that iontophoresis and phonophoresis of naproxen are equally effective electrotherapy methods in the treatment of lateral epicondylitis [60].

Demirtaş et al., suggest positive effect of iontophoresis in the treatment of lateral epicondylitis and indicate that iontophoresis of sodium diclofenac is more effective than that of sodium salicylate [61].

The effectiveness of this therapeutic method has also been tested in secondary painful events in arthritic disease of the spine. Patients were treated with diclofenac sodium and betamethasone for 20 minutes and evaluated immediately after the end of the treatment and after 24 hours, by detecting a significant reduction of spontaneous pain after the application, which is maintained unchanged even at 24 hours [62]. Also in subjects with inflammatory disease, iontophoresis returns excellent results, as observed in subjects with inserted pes anserine bursitis in a study, the purpose of which was to compare the efficacy of conventional oral therapy with anti-inflammatory, mesotherapy and (Isofor Compact) electroporation using the same substance. In all groups, we were obtained with similar results in terms of decrease in pain and improvement in quality of life at the end of the third week of treatment. However, the ultrasonography showed a hypoechoic area reduction of pes anserine bursitis only in the groups treated with mesotherapy and electroporation [63].

Moreover, iontophoresis appears a safe and applicable method in a complex rehabilitation project, also in children, as in the case of osteochondrosis of the tibial tuberosity, inflammatory degenerative disease. The results showed a significant reduction in pain even after the first two weeks of treatment and pain relief in its third week. A significant improvement in the ultrasound examination at the end of the protocol with normalization of the patellar tendon thickness and peritendinous edema resorption, a symmetrization of the load at podobarometric examination and a significant improvement in the isokinetic test [64].

5. Phonoforesis

Another interesting method of treatment of Psychiatric and Rehabilitation Medicine is the phonophoresis, that consists in the use of ultrasound for transcutaneous drug delivery.

Cutaneous bioavailability in most of the marketed dermatological formulations is low.

The skin represents a significant barrier to the entrance of foreign substances, but is also a potential therapeutic away.

The stratum corneum has a structure in determining barrier function. The corneocytes (about 85% of the mass of the stratum corneum) and intercellular lipids (15%) are arranged in about 15–20 layers [65]. It consists of approximately: 70% protein, 15% lipids, and only 15% of water [66]. In corneocytes, thickened keratin and filaggrin and cleavage products are present. The corneocytes is rich in protein and is surrounded by lipids [67]. Weight ratio of 50% ceramides, 35–40% cholesterol, fatty acids liberi10–15% contained within the extracellular spaces and arranged in double layer slats make the stratum corneum impermeable to water soluble substances [68].

Changes of this lamellar structure and/or of its lipid composition constitute the biochemist and structural basis of permeability variations related to the body site.

It is possible to increase the penetration of active substances through the stratum corneum using ultrasound, reaching, thus, the area to be treated with the appropriate concentration of drug at a certain depth and in a selective way, without dispersion in bloodstream and first pass effect [69]. Ultrasound (US) produces alterations in the structure of the stratum corneum and increases the permeability [70]. (**Figure 9**)

Temperature increase induced by the US increases the kinetic energy of drug's molecules, dilates the points of entry through the skin (hair follicles and sweat glands), and increases the blood flow in the treated area [71]. US also produce mechanical effects as microstreming and cavitation of cells, or in any case nonthermal effects as reduction of the membrane potential, alterations of lipid structure, with increased cell permeability and ionic conductance [72].

Cavitation refers to the formation and collapse of small air bubbles formed in a liquid due to a pressure change induced in the tissue fluid from the passage of ultrasound. (**Figure 10 a - b**)

Cavitation can be stable (when ultrasound of high intensity and low frequency passing through a liquid, produce small bubbles that oscillate rhythmically in size) or unstable (when high-frequency ultrasound generate bubbles that grow and collapse abruptly). (**Figure 10 c - d**)

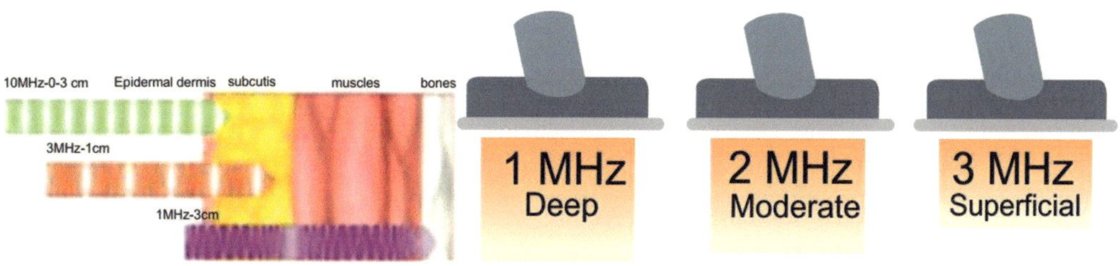

Figure 9. Ultrsound characteristics.

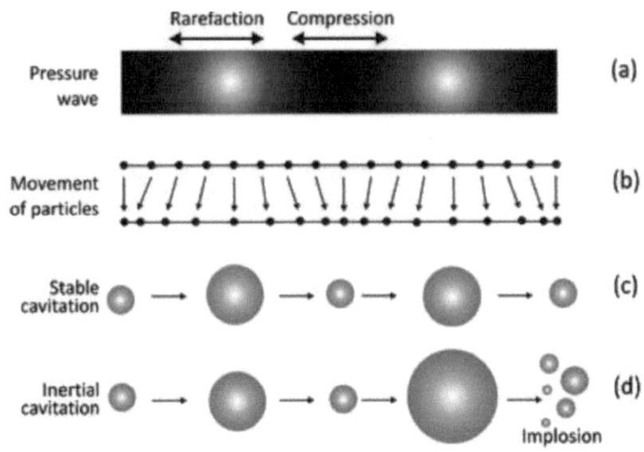

Figure 10. Cavitation phenomenon.

For microstreaming, it means the formation of vortices in small volumes of cytoplasmic and interstitial fluid; this improves the dissolution of the drug particles in suspension and alters the cell membrane structure by setting the permeability to sodium and calcium ions [73].

For a long time, effective frequencies have been investigated to produce therapeutic effect.

Ultrasound for therapeutic purposes, are used in physical and rehabilitation medicine with a range between 0.75 and 3 MHz: lower frequencies penetrate most deeply (3–5 cm) and are preferred in subjects with a high percentage of body fat, while higher frequencies are absorbed from superficial tissues (1–2 cm) (**Figure 11**).

In rehabilitation, phonophoresis is used to convey drugs such as corticosteroids and NSAIDs to treat diseases affecting the musculoskeletal system, such as osteoarthritis treated by Boyaci et al. with 100 mg of ketoprofen using an applicator 5 cm in diameter, with a frequency of 1 MHz, with a power of 1.5 W/cm^2 for 8 min. Patients involved in the study were assessed before and after treatment with VAS scale, 15-m walking time, and Western Ontario and McMaster Universities Arthritis Index (WOMAC), and reported a significant improvement in their condition [74]. Also a study of Tascioglu et al. showed greater efficacy of pulsed mode than continuous mode in the treatment of osteoarthritis of the knee [75].

Luksurapan has instead used 20 mg of piroxicam in continuous mode, power, 1.0 W/cm^2 in sessions from 10 minutes to treat the same disease, obtaining excellent results in particular relating to the VAS scale [76].

Another disease that can be treated with phonophoresis is the painful myofascial syndrome, treated with diclofenac gel (Voltaren emulgel) applied with an applicator 5 cm in diameter at 1 MHz of frequency and power 1.5 W/cm^2 for 10 minutes on two trigger points of the trapezius muscle, with improvement in pain compared to the baseline condition [77].

For temporomandibular joint (TMJ) pain phonophoresis with 1.0 MHz frequency, power 0.8 to 1.5 W/cm^2 in continuous mode for 15 minutes was applied, with results suggesting that transdermal delivery of indomethacin with US has significant effect on the TMJ pain [78].

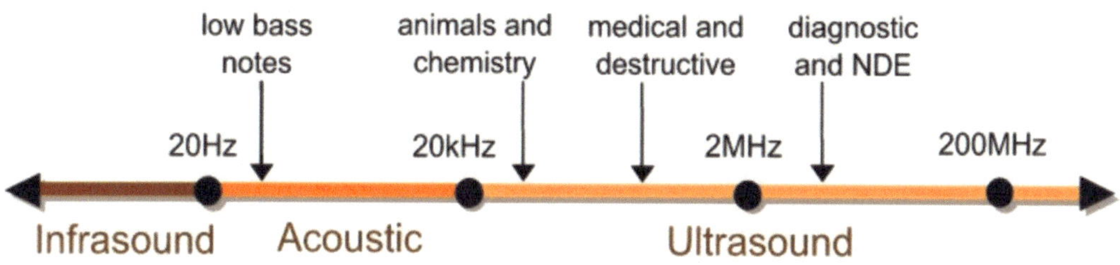

Figure 11. Frequencies of ultrasound and application area.

Another experience is related to use of phonophoresis with ultrasound of high intensity and low frequency passing through the skin (hair follicles and sweat glands) with addition of an anti-inflammatory phytotherapy gel in treatment of Biceps Long Head tendinitis in rotator cuff disease compared to a Extracorporeal Shock Wave Therapy (ESWT) treatment of the rotator cuff tendinitis.

At the present time, there are no specific and standard protocols for the application of ultrasound to the transdermal drug delivery, because of multiple variables of treatment such as frequency, method of delivery, molecular structure of the drug, patients' age, thickness, and hydration of the skin.

It is definitely a treatment that offers advantages compared to the oral administration of anti-inflammatories.

Despite the contradictions in the various studies on mode of administration, frequency and drug use, almost all agree on the effectiveness of this therapeutic method in relieving pain and restoration of function that is impaired in different conditions affecting the musculoskeletal system [74].

6. Phytotherapy

Acute and chronic diseases of the musculoskeletal system represent about 40% of health demands. If you add to this the progressive increase in the average lifespan resulting in increased incidence of mechanical, metabolic and consumption alterations, that are the basis of chronic myofascial and joints' diseases, it understands the interest toward an "complementary medicine." In this context, phytotherapy and the search for natural substances that act on inflammation and pain fit perfectly.

Inflammation is a response model to the damage; it leads to accumulation of cells and exudates in tissues harmed in to protect from further damage. Inflammation has been studied for thousands years to try to counteract the effects it has on the human body [79].

Phytotherapy is the use of plant-derived medications in the treatment or prevention of more inflammatory and noninflammatory diseases. Indeed medical herbalism which is characterized by an empirical approach, phytotherapy is a science-based medical practice. Numerous trials and pharmacological studies of specific phytotherapeutic preparations exist. In some countries, it is considered sufficient to license phytotherapeutic products as medicines, whereas in other countries, phytotherapy is viewed as a form of traditional medicines.

The concept of phytotherapy was originated by French physician Henri Leclerc, who first used the term in 1913 and who published various editions of the Précis de phytothérapie the first in 1922. Successively, in 1934, the term Phytotherapy was used in common as a definition by Eric Frederick William Powell, an English expert of herbalism. Only in 1960, a German herbalist and physician Rudolf Fritz Weiss published Lehrbuch der Phytotherapie (1960; Herbal Medicine), which determined a definition of this topic in all Europe [80].

Only in the 1980s, the scientific research published in scientific article (as in journal Phytotherapy Research) with a definition in the medical-scientific field of phytotherapy began.

A commonly used in phytotherapy is standardization, which is the need to have a minimum of one or more active compounds or groups of plant extract compounds.

Natural products with anti-inflammatory activity have long been used as a folk remedy for inflammatory conditions such as fever, pain, migraine, and arthritis. The report of the British Nutrition Foundation offers a classification of phytochemicals useful information on products with anti-inflammatory properties [81].

Extensive scientific research revealed that curcumin has anti-inflammatory action [82].

The anti-inflammatory activity of curcumin is mainly due to the inhibition of arachidonic acid metabolism, cyclooxygenase (COX), lipoxygenase (LOX), interleukin (IL), tumor necrosis factor (TNF) and also due to the stabilization of the lysosomal membrane [83–85].

In the pathogenesis of arthritis sundry inflammatory cytokines (TNF, IL-1, IL-6), phlogosis enzymes (COX-2, 5-LOX, MMP-9) and adhesion molecules have a central role and almost all of this are synthesized following the gene transcription of NF-kB. Joe et al. investigated the effect of curcumin on acid glycoprotein in serum of rats with induced arthritis [86]. Treating inflammation in these rats with arthritis induced with curcumin per os, has been seen a 73% reduction in the levels of Gp A72.

The typical cartilage consumption that occurs in rheumatoid arthritis, is due to the action of matrix metalloproteinases (MMPs), whose MMP-1 and MMP-3 genes are over expressed in synovial fibroblasts of patients affected by this disease rheumatoid arthritis. Onodera et al. [87] have shown that curcumin blocks the upregulation of MMP mRNA.

Furthermore, curcumin can enhance the growth inhibitory and pro-apoptotic effects of celecoxib in synovial cells in OA as noted by Lev-Ari et al [88]. A synergistic effect was observed in the inhibition of cell growth when the cells were exposed to celecoxib combined with curcumin. The inhibitory effect of the combination of these drugs on cell growth resulted in an increase of apoptosis induction. The use of celecoxib at lower concentrations and more secure in combination with curcumin can provide a combination of novel treatment for OA and other rheumatologic disorders.

To relieve symptoms of arthritis is also used Lyprinol, extracted from green mussels from New Zealand, containing triglycerides, sterols, polar lipids and free fatty acids. Lyprinol showed a significant anti-inflammatory activity in induced polyarthritis in rats [89]. The mechanism by which the lyprinolo acts remains unclear. It certainly reduce proinflammatory LTB4 in human monocytes. Additionally, a human study showed that NZGLM reduces levels of TXB2, PGE2 and IL-1β with a similar power to low doses of omega-3 supplement [90].

The first natural substance used as anti-inflammatory in rheumatoid arthritis and osteoarthritis, was bromelain in 1964 [91]. It is an aqueous extract obtained from stem and fruit of the Pineapple plant. It has several beneficial effects, including the reversible inhibition of platelet aggregation. Currently, it is used mainly in acute inflammation and sports injuries. The anti-inflammatory mechanism is due to increasing serum fibrinolytic activity, reduction in plasma fibrinogen levels, decreasing levels of PGE2, TXA2, reduction in bradykinin levels with subsequent reduction in vascular permeability and thus edema; and modulating the adhesion molecules of the immune system cells.

In the treatment of muscle damage, Arnica is also widely used; also known as mountain daisy, mountain tobacco, and leopard's bane, Arnica is a perennial herb of the family Asteraceae [92].

Lyss et al. demonstrated that helenalin, the most active compound from Arnica, inhibits the transcription factor nuclear factor kappa B (NF-kB) through the alteration and stabilization of NF-kB/inhibitor of kappa B complex (IkappaB) in cells T, B cells and epithelial cells and abolish the expression of kappa B gene-driven. Later work showed that helenalin can inhibit the migration and chemotaxis of human neutrophils and activities of 5-lipoxygenase and leukotriene C4 synthase. As Lyss et al. postulated in 1997, Helenalin indirectly reduces the expression of NF-kB, acting on expression of surface receptors CD25, CD28, CD27, and CD120b that, if occupied, transduce the activation signal for NF-kB [93].

The activation of NF-kB promotes the release of proinflammatory cytokines and the recruitment of local leukocytes, generating pain and phlogosis.

The Arnica ability to inhibit the activation of NF-kB nuclear transcription factors of activated T cells and pro-inflammatory cytokines IL-1b TNF-a are related with their contents, quantity, and quality of sesquiterpene lactones.

When you consider that muscle damage induced by exercise and delayed onset muscles soreness (DOMS) are accompanied by a systemic inflammatory response that is responsible for initiating, amplifying and/or resolving of muscle damage, one can understand why arnica has a role in these situations.

Overall, Arnica (topical and/or oral formulations) showed reproducible clinical benefits, some of which are comparable with anti-inflammatory drugs such as diclofenac [93], ibuprofen, and corticosteroids [94], which are considered the therapy of choice for the treatment of osteoarthritis, postoperative edema, and bruising [95].

The Arnica topical use is supported by studies that prove its effectiveness in reducing the acute muscle pain induced by exercise,[96, 97] and in the symptomatic treatment of osteoarthritis.

Local action is exerted on the muscle, calming the sensation of pain; in the joints, reducing the swelling and pain caused by rheumatic diseases; on the vascular district, reducing hematoma and bruising and protecting blood vessels.

7. Homeopathy

Homeopathy, from the greek ὅμοιος, omoios, "similar" and πάθος, pathos, "suffering," was developed in the late 700s by a German doctor, Samuel Hahnemann, in an age when the symptoms were cured with "therapies" often more lethal than diseases, such as bloodletting and enemas. Hahnemann was convinced that the same substance at high doses cause a disease in healthy people, instead, at infnitesimal doses could cure sick people. Also he claimed that diluting especially substances ("potentiation" obtained by the succession of serial dilutions) not only reduced or abolished the toxic effect, but also, paradoxically, increased their curative power [98]. Homeopathy is a pharmaceutical preparation that contains, in equal parts, different homeopathic dilutions prepared from the same tincture [99]. In Italy, homeopathy is regulated by normative reference for homeopathy Legislative Decree of 24 April 2006, no. 219 "Implementation of Directive 2001/83/EC (and subsequent amending Directives) on a Community code relating to medicinal products for human use, as well as the Directive 2003/94/EC. For preparing a homeopathic diluition, in fact, one starts from a basic substance which is then diluted and dynamized. A critical step is the preparation of the mother tincture, whose production technique is described in the French Official Pharmacopoeia (X edition 1983). The ratio between the dried product and water-alcohol mixture is 1:10. The degree of water-alcohol mixture varies in relation to the solubility of the products to be extracted: a plant with predominantly water-soluble active substances is lower with respect to the title of a substance with principles less water-soluble active. It will have to macerate for 21 days, while for an alcoholic tincture it takes 5–10 days. The effects of homeopathic medicines have been studied in numerous study with experimental inflammation [100–103] Homeopathic clinical research has developed over the last twenty years with the increasingly greater use of modern medical methods (clinical trials, observational studies, statistic evaluations, computerized storage programs and instrumental or laboratory testing). For example, *Atropa belladonna* (Belladonna) is commonly used for treatment of local inflammation: it is prescribed for reducing severe pain, inflammation or any infection, especially on the upper part of the respiratory tract. Belladonna is most suitable to treat disorders of the heart, blood vessels, lungs as well as the neuropathic pain. The toxic juice of *Atropa belladonna* in homeopathic formulation is extremely diluted with alcohol in order to eliminate even the slightest trace of toxicity and to remove harmfulness. This procedure makes it suitable for human use [104, 105].

There are three extracts of *Echinacea*: *E. pallida, E. angustifolia,* and *E. purpurea* that are proposed as phytoimmunostimulating agents and their activity is mainly directed toward the nonspecific cellular immune system [106] Echinacea angustifolia that is used for many years also in traditional medicine, acts in determining an increase of leukocyte activity, stimulation of phagocytosis, TNF production by macrophages and increase of T and B cell activity, as well as gINF production by lymphocytes [107]. Furthermore, *Echinacea* has antioxidant effects and free radical scavenging capacities, related to the content in polyphenolic compounds. Echinacoside, chlorogenic acid, chicoric acid, cynarine and caffeic acid inhibit the production of free radicals and lipid peroxidation, classic inflammation consequence. All of this caffeoyl derived, are contained in *Echinacea*. Besides, echinacoside induce degradation of type III collagen with a potential role in cicatrizacion and fibrosys treatment [108]. A series of step-by-step research trial about the biological effects of homeopathic Arnica montana, specially the Arnica montana 6cH, using animal models is presented in literature [109]. Arnica montana is a plant from the family Compositae native of East and Central Europe hills. Leaves, flowers, and roots contain tannins, flavonoids, lactones sesquirterpenic, alcohols and obviously helenalin which is the active principle best known [110]. It acts inhibiting the transcription factor NFκβ, like a corticoid steroids [111]. Trauma pain and oedema absorption are the main indications for the clinical and experimental use of this homeopathic preparation [94, 112–115].

Others studies show that Arnica montana 6cH is able to modulate the acute inflammatory process in rats, since it can increase lymphatic oedema absorption and local blood flow, as well as to promote the array of polymorphonuclear cell migration [116]. Four homeopathic remedies can be used for arthritis: causticum (6cH, 30cH) typically helpful in rheumatoid arthritis, this remedy is known for its anti-inflammatory action on the muscles, tendons, and nerves; calcarea carbonica (6cH, 30cH), this remedy has many disorders associated with calcium metabolism and is helpful in many cases of osteoarthritis; colchicum can be used for rheumatoid arthritis and gout for controlling pains in the small joints, especially the big toe, and minimal swelling; nux vomica (6cH, 30cH) in joint pains, especially in the knees [117].

These are only a few of the hundreds of homeopathic remedies that can be helpful in inflammatory conditions.

8. Topical application

The human epidermal permeabilities of different NSAIDs (salicylic acid, diethylamine salicylate, indomethacin, naproxen, diclofenac and piroxicam) from aqueous solutions is dependent on the drug's lipophilicity [118]. Topical application can be applied over the site of injury or pain area like lumbar or cervical zone and its analgesic and anti-inflammatory effects are expressed in the underlying superficial or musculoskeletal soft tissue. This modality of administration of NSAIDs acts locally and is not dependent on systemic absorption and subsequent redistribution into peripheral tissues with significantly lower systemic side effects Furthermore, it is a direct access and it allows prolonged use above all in patients who cannot use no oral medications [95, 119–120]. Of the available formulations is the epolamine salt of diclofenac that offers specific advantages for topical administration. The surfactant property of diclofenac epolamine improves hydration of the stratum corneum so it increases surface tension at the interface between the skin and the topical pharmaceutical preparation, favouring absorption [121]. Diclofenac epolamine topical patch is indicated for treatment of acute pain of minor strains, sprains, and contusions and as a home therapy in a complex rehabilitation project in soft tissue diseases (e.g., tendonitis, epicondylitis), or rheumatologic disorders (e.g., osteoarthritis, rheumatoid arthritis), or extra-articular pathologies (e.g., fibrositis). Each adhesive patch contains 180 mg of diclofenac epolamine and inactive excipients, which enhance skin hydration and facilitate plaster adherence. Following the application of diclofenac twice daily for 5 days, were found peak plasma concentrations of 0.7–6.0 ng/mL at 10–20 hours. In the bloodstream, diclofenac has a half-life of about 12 hours and it is widely linked to albumin [122]. Its metabolism is urinary and biliary excretion of the sulfate and glucuronide conjugates. In 19 clinical trials, tolerability and efficacy of the various topical formulations of diclofenac (1.5% diclofenac sodium solution, 1.16% diclofenac diethylamine gel, 140 mg diclofenac hydroxyethylpyrrolidine patch, and 2% diclofenac lecithin organogel) have been recently revised, whereas approximately 3000 patients treated [123]. Furthermore, Diclofenac sodium 1% gel is used commonly for the relief of pain due to osteoarthritis such as the knees and those of the hands. This product contains a variety of additional ingredients in the vehicle including isopropyl alcohol, propylene glycol, and water to assist in drug penetration of the skin [124]. Topical administration is linked to local skin irritation or allergies [125].

Mg^{2+} may be one of these components because it has a significant role in energy metabolism via basic mitochondrial function, ATP transmembrane transport, muscle contraction or relaxation, membrane stability, and neuromuscular, cardiovascular, immune and hormonal functions [126–129]. Mg^{2+} depletion has been reported to decrease antioxidant capacity, increase oxidative stress, and impair intracellular calcium homeostasis that result in swelling and structural damage to muscle cells [130].

Some study shows that transdermal application may be better accepted than oral application in these patients with fibromyalgia for control of pain and inflammation because it is usually used a multitude of oral medications. Transdermal $MgCl_2$ solution is ideal for use in transdermal applications because it is rapidly absorbed through the skin and, therefore, can rapidly increase low or depleted levels of magnesium in the body [31, 131]. Engen et al suggest that transdermal Mg Cl_2 applied twice daily (16 sprays of $MgCl_2$ which equals 400 mg of magnesium) on the upper and lower limbs may be beneficial for patients with fibromyalgia [132].

9. Galenic formulations

A new galenic formulation has recently been developed. Galenic formulations with lower treatment burdens are associated with better patient compliance and persistence compared with older more burdensome modalities. Galenic formulations are characterized by low cost of the production system and the simple operative procedures; the possibility to adapt dosages and pharmaceutical forms to the patients' needs and medical prescriptions; reduction in the use of counterfeit medicines in the settings where the Galenic laboratories are located [133]. It is a therapeutic aspect evolving, so it requires others studies over the next few years.

10. Conclusion

This chapter gives an overview about the state of the art regarding the use of NSAIDs in physical and rehabilitation medicine, not only used by the classical routes of administration, but especially about the uses of these drugs through own means of this branch of medicine.

Author details

Rosa Grazia Bellomo[1], Simona Maria Carmignano[2], Tommaso Palermo[2], Lucia Cosenza[2], Andrea Saggini[3] and Raoul Saggini[4]*

*Address all correspondence to: saggini@unich.it

1 Department of Medical Sciences, Oral and Biotechnology, "G. d'Annunzio" University, Chieti, Italy

2 School of Specialties in PRM, "G. d'Annunzio" University, Chieti, Italy

3 Department of Biomedicine and Prevention, Institute of Anatomic Pathology, University of Rome Tor Vergata, Rome, Italy

4 Department of Medical Sciences, Oral and Biotechnology, "G. d'Annunzio" University, Chieti, Italy

References

[1] Weiss U. Inflammation. Nature. 2008;**454**(7203):427. DOI: 10.1038/454427a

[2] Medzhitov R. Origin and physiological roles of inflammation. Nature. 2008;**454**(7203): 428-435. DOI: 10.1038/nature07201

[3] Akira S, Uematsu S, Takeuchi O. Pathogen recognition and innate immunity. Cell. 2006;**124**(4):783-801. DOI: 10.1016/j.cell.2006.02.015

[4] Zhu CB, Blakely RD, Hewlett WA. The proinflammatory cytokines interleukin-1beta and tumor necrosis factor-alpha activate serotonin transporters. Neuropsychopharmacology. 2006;**31**(10):2121-2131. DOI: 10.1038/sj.npp.1301029

[5] Ding W, Stohl LL, Wagner JA, Granstein RD. Calcitonin gene-related peptide biases Langerhans cells toward Th2-type immunity. Journal of Immunology. 2008;**181**:6020-6026

[6] Sauer SK, Reeh PW, Bove GM. Noxious heat-induced CGRP release from rat sciatic nerve axons in vitro. The European Journal of Neuroscience. 2001;**14**:1203-1208

[7] McMahon, Bennet. Bevan's Wall and Melzack's Textbook of Pain. Elsevier Churchill Livingstone. London. 2006;49-72

[8] Alfred IT. Metchnikoff and the phagocytosis theory. Nature Reviews Molecular Cell Biology. 2003;**4**:897-901. DOI: 10.1038/nrm1244

[9] Christopher DB, Derek WG, and Charles NS. Pro-resolving lipid mediators and mechanisms in the resolution of acute inflammation. Immunity. 2014;**40**(3):315-327. DOI: 10.1016/j.immuni.2014.02.009

[10] Serhan CN, Savill J. Resolution of inflammation: The beginning programs the end. Nature Immunology. 2005;**6**(12):1191-1197. DOI: 10.1038/ni1276

[11] Hotamisligil GS. Inflammation and metabolic disorders. Nature. 2006;**444**(7121):860-867. DOI: 10.1038/nature05485

[12] Hawkey CJ. COX-2 inhibitors. Lancet. 1999;**15**:307-314. DOI: 10.1016/S0140-6736(98)12154-2

[13] Brooks PM, Day RO. Nonsteroidal antiinflammatory drugs—differences and similarities. The New England Journal of Medicine. 1991;**324**(24):1716-1725. DOI: 10.1056/NEJM199106133242407

[14] Berde C, Sundel R. COX 2 Inhibitors: A Status Report [Internet]. 1998. Available from: www.iasp-pain.org/TC98SeptOct.html

[15] Antman EM, Bennett JS, Daugherty A. Use of nonsteroidal antiinflammatory drugs: an update for clinicians: A scientific statement from the American Heart Association. Circulation. 2007;**115**(12):1634-1642. DOI: 10.1161/CIRCULATIONAHA.106.181424

[16] World Health Organization. Cancer Pain Relief with a Guide to Opioid Availability. 2nd ed. Geneva; 1996. 15-16

[17] Stöllberger C, Finsterer J. Nonsteroidal anti-inflammatory drugs in patients with cardio- or cerebrovascular disorders. Zeitschrift für Kardiologie. 2003;**92**(9):721-729. DOI: 10.1007/s00392-003-0964-x

[18] Dalloz-Bourguignon A. A new therapy against pain: Mesotherapy (author's transl). Journal Belge de Médecine Physique et de Réhabilitation 1979;**2**:230-234

[19] Pistor M. What is mesotherapy?. Le Chirurgien-Dentiste de France. 1976;**46**(288):59-60

[20] Vecchiet L, Giamberardino MA, Saggini R. Myofascial pain syndromes: Clinical and pathophysiological aspects. Clinical Journal of Pain. 1991;**1**:S16-S22

[21] Saggini R, Bellomo RG, Cancelli F, Iodice P. Treatment on myofascial pain syndromes: Local acoustic vibration vs local lidocaine. Journal of Rehabilitation Medicine. 2007;1650-1977

[22] Brinks A, van Rijn RM, Willemsen SP. Corticosteroid injections for greater trochanteric pain syndrome: A randomized controlled trial in primary care. Annals of Family Medicine. 2011;**9**(3):226-234. DOI: 10.1370/afm.1232

[23] Marcelli S. Nuovo Manuale di Mesoterapia.Ed. Milano: Ulrico Hoepli; 2013. chapt.4

[24] Ruggeri F, Bartoletti CA, Maggiori S. Clinical results of the multicentric experimentation. Giornale di Mesoterapia. 1981;**1**:47-49

[25] Colombo I, Cigolini M, Combi F. Clinical results of the multicentric experimentation. Giornale di Mesoterapia. 1981;**1**:50-52

[26] Saraceni VPalieri G, De Pedis M. Clinical results of the multicentric experimentation. Giornale di Mesoterapia. 1981;**1**:53-59

[27] Piantoni D Cotichelli E, Di Gianvito P. Clinical results of the multicentric experimentation. Giornale di Mesoterapia. 1981;**1**:60-63

[28] Pezone A, Villa L, Martini D. Clinical results of the multicentric experimentation. Giornale di Mesoterapia. 1981;**1**:64-66

[29] Curro F, Bearzato A. Use of the S-adenosil l-methionine ` (Same) in the treatment of degenerative arthropathies of arthrosis. Nature. 1981;**1**:99-107

[30] Guazzetti R, Iotti E, Marinoni E. Mesotherapy with naproxin sodium in musculoskeletal diseases. Rivista Europea Per Le Scienze Mediche E Farmacologiche. 1988;**10**:539-542

[31] Narvarte DA, Rosset-Llobet J. Safety of subcutaneous microinjections (mesotherapy) in musicians. Medical Problems of Performing Artists. 2011;**2**:79-83

[32] Capone M, Stancati MT, Tolla V, Chiatti R, Muscolo V, Pasquale M. Observations on the administration of sodium edetate in calcified scapulohumeral periarthritis. Ionophoresis and mesotherapy: Comparison of two techniques. Ortopedia e Traumatologia Oggi. 1994;**14**:163-168

[33] Piantoni D, Cotichellil E, Santilli W. Use of calcitonin in regional osteoporosis. Giornale di Mesoterapia. 1985;**5**:21-23

[34] Curro F, Bearzatto A. Mesotherapy in the treatment of `post-zoster neuritis. Giornale di Mesoterapia. 1985;**5**:37-43

[35] Curro F, Bearzatto A, Fontanini C. Mesotherapy in a general medicine department: A year of activity. Giornale diMesoterapia. 1983;**3**:25-28

[36] Pezone A, Santuari E, Villa ML et al. The distinct analgesicaction of calcitonin in treating painful diseases of joints with mesotherapy. Giornale di Mesoterapia. 1986;**6**:19-23

[37] Romano M, Marcone E, Concetta Meo M, Attanasio L. Orgotein: Our experience in rheumatic pathology. Giornale di Mesoterapia. 1985;**5**:25-28

[38] Solinas G, Solinas AL, Perra P, Solinas FL. Treatment of mechanical tendinopathies by mesotherapy with orgotein in combination with laser therapy. Riabilitazione. 1987;**4**:281-288

[39] Garzya G, Leucci PF, Greco T, Branca L, Moschettini V. Comparative stydy of three non-steroid anti-inflammatory drugs used with mesotherapy techique in 100 geriatric patients affected by muscular -skeletal pathology. Giornale di Mesoterapia. 1987;**7**:31-44

[40] Di Cesare A, Giombini A, Di Cesare M, Ripani M, Vulpiani MC, Saraceni VM. Comparison between the effects of trigger point mesotherapy versus acupuncture points mesotherapy in the treatment of chronic low back pain: A short term randomized controlled trial. Complementary Therapies in Medicine. 2011;**19**:19-26

[41] Costantino C, Marangio E, Coruzzi G. Mesotherapy versus systemic therapy in the treatment of acute low back pain: A randomized trial. Evidence-based Complementary and Alternative Medicine. 2011;**2011**. pii: 317183. DOI: 10.1155/2011/317183

[42] Saggini R, Di Stefano A, Dodaj I, Scarcello L, Bellomo RG. Pes anserine bursitis in symptomatic osteoarthritis patients: A mesotherapy treatment study. Journal of Alternative and Complementary Medicine. 2015;**21**(8):480-484. DOI: 10.1089/acm.2015.0007

[43] Rawat S, Vengurlekar S, Rakesh B. Transdermal delivery by iontophoresis. Indian Journal of Pharmaceutical Sciences. 2008;**70**(1):5-10

[44] Helmstädter A. The history of electrically-assisted transdermal drug delivery ("iontophoresis"). Pharmazie. 2001;**56**:583-587

[45] Burton H, Sage JR. Iontophoresis. Maibach, HI, editors. In: Percutaneous Penetration Enhancers. Boca Raton, FL, USA: CRC Press; 1995. 351-367

[46] Pikal MJ. The role of electroosmosic flow in transdermal iontophoresis. Advanced Drug Delivery Reviews. 2001;**46**(1-3):281-305

[47] Kanikkannan N. Iontophoresis based transdermal delivery systems. Biodrugs. 2002; **16**:339-347

[48] Hu QH, Liang WQ. A comparative study of electroporation and iontophoresis for percutaneous penetration of naproxen. Pharmazie. 2003;**58**(3):192-194

[49] Guy RH, Hadgraft J. Rate control in transdermal drug delivery?. International Journal of Pharmaceutics 1992;**82**(3):DOI: 10.1016/0378-5173(92)90183-3

[50] Fang J, et al. Passive and iontophoretic delivery of three diclofenac salts across various skin types. Biological & Pharmaceutical Bulletin. 2000;**23**(11):1357-1362

[51] Hui X et al. Pharmacokinetic and local tissue disposition of sodium diclofenac following iontophoresis and systemic administration in rabbits. Journal of Pharmaceutical Sciences. 2001;**90**(9):1269-1276

[52] Gay CL, et al. Iontophoretic delivery of piroxicam across the skin in vitro. Journal of Controlled Release. 1992;**22**(1):57-67

[53] Curdy C, et al. Piroxicam delivery into human stratum corneum in vivo: Iontophoresis versus passive diffusion. Journal of Controlled Release. 2001;**76**(1-2):73-79

[54] Tiwari SB, Udupa N. Investigation into the potential of iontophoresis facilitated delivery of ketorolac. International Journal of Pharmaceutics. 2003;**260**(1):93-103

[55] Garagiola U, et al. Iontophoretic administration of pirprofen or lysine soluble aspirin in the treatment of rheumatic diseases. Clinical Therapeutics. 1998;**10**(5):553-558

[56] Grossi E, et al. NSAID ionisation in the management of soft-tissue rheumatism: Role played by the drug, electrical stimulation and suggestion. Clinical and Experimental Rheumatology. 1986;**4**(3):265-267

[57] Vecchini L, Grossi E. Ionization with diclofenac sodium in rheumatic disorders: A double-blind placebo-controlled trial. Journal of International Medical Research. 1984;**12**(6):346-350

[58] Famaey JP, et al. Ionisation with Voltaren. A multi-centre trial. Journal Belge de Médecine Physique et de Réhabilitation. 1982; **5**(2):55-60

[59] Saggini R, Zoppi M, Vecchiet F, Gatteschi L, Obletter G. Comparison of electromotive drug administration with ketorolac or with placebo in patients with pain from rheumatic disease: A double-masked study. Clinical Therapeutics. 1996;**18**(6):1169-1174

[60] Baskurt F, Ozean A, Algún C. Comparison of effects of phonophoresis and iontophoresis of naproxen in the treatment of lateral epicondylitis. Clinical Rehabilitation. 2003;**17**:96-100

[61] Demirtaş RN, Oner C. The treatment of lateral epicondylitis by iontophoresis of sodium salicylate and sodium diclofenac. Clinical Rehabilitation. 1998;**12**(1):23-29

[62] Lerza R, Fabrizio A, Savini A, Affaitati G, Bellomo RG, Saggini R. Effects of hydroelectrophoresis (Hydrofor) on articular pain. Dolore: Aggiornamenti Clinici. 2009;**1-2**(S):116-117

[63] Saggini R, D' Ettole S, Ancona E, Barassi G, Bellomo RG et al. Borsite della zampa d'oca in pazienti con gonartrosi: Studio sulla veicolazione transdermica isoforetica. conference proceedings 43° Congresso Nazionale SIMFER Ferrara 2015

[64] Bellomo RG, Carmignano S, Ancona E, Barassi G, Saggini R. Il dolore anteriore di ginocchio in età pediatrica: dalla valutazione al tratamento sicuro ed efcace con precoce ripresa funzionale. Giornale italiano di medicina riabilitativa. Edizioni Minerva Medica. Volume 29 N. 2/3 Agosto-Dicembre 2015 Roma

[65] Walters KA, Roberts MS. The structure and function of skin. Walters KA, editors. In: Dermatological and Transdermal Formulations. New York: Marcel Dekker; 2002. 1-40

[66] Berardesca E, Rona C. Barriera cutanea e farmaci. In: Tratato di Dermatologia. Padova: Piccin; Padova 2007. pp. 1-12

[67] Lampe MA, Burlingame AL, Whitney J, Williams ML, Brown BE, et al. Human stratum corneum lipids: Characterization and regional differences. Journal of Lipid Research. 1983;**24**:120-130

[68] Elias PM, Menon GK. Structural and lipid biochemical correlates of the epidermal permeability barrier. Advances in Lipid Research. 1991;**24**:1-26

[69] Kassan DG, Lynch AM, Stiller MJ. Physical enhancement of dermatologic drug delivery: Iontophoresis and phonophoresis. Journal of the American Academy of Dermatology. 1996;**34**:657-666

[70] Merino G, Kalia YN, Guy RH. Ultrasound-enhanced transdermal transport. Journal of Pharmaceutical Sciences. 2003;**92**:1125-1137

[71] Dinno MA, Dyson M, Young SR, et al. The significance of membrane changes in the safe and effective use of therapeutic and diagnostic ultrasound. Ultrasound in Medicine & Biology. 1989;**34**:1543-1552

[72] Nyborg WL. Mechanisms. Nyborg WL, Ziskin MC, editors. In: Biological Effects of Ultrasound. New York, NY: Churchill Livingstone Inc; 1985:23-33

[73] Byl NN. The use of ultrasound as an enhancer for transcutaneous drug delivery: Phonophoresis. Physical Therapy. 1995;**75**(6):539-553

[74] Boyaci A. Comparison of the efficacy of ketoprofen phonophoresis, ultrasound, and short-wave diathermy in knee osteoarthritisAhmet. Rheumatology International. 2013;**33**:2811-2818

[75] Tascioglu F, Kuzgun S, Armagan O, Ogutler G. Short-term effectiveness of ultrasound therapy in knee osteoarthritis. The Journal of International Medical Research. 2010;**38**(4):1233-1242

[76] Luksurapan W, Boonhong J. Effects of phonophoresis of piroxicam and ultrasound on symptomatic knee osteoarthritis. Archives of Physical Medicine and Rehabilitation. 2013;**94**:250-255

[77] Ay S, Doğan SK, Evcik D, Başer OC. Comparison the efficacy of phonophoresis and ultrasound therapy in myofascial pain syndrome. Rheumatology International. 2011;**31**:1203-1208. DOI: 10.1007/s00296-010-1419-0

[78] Shin SM, Choi JK. Effect of indomethacin phonophoresis on the relief of temporomandibular joint pain. Cranio. 1997;**15**:345-348

[79] Gaofeng Y. Natural products and anti-inflammatory activity. Asia Pacific Journal of Clinical Nutrition. 2006;**15** (2):143-152

[80] Weiss RF. In: Weiss's Herbal Medicine. Stoccarda: Classic Edition Thieme; Stoccarda 2001

[81] Golberg G. Plants: Diet and Health. The Report of a British Nutrition Foundation Task Force. British Nutrition Foundation, Blackwell Publishing. 2003; 1-26. DOI: 10.1002/9780470774465

[82] Satoskar RR, Shah SJ, Shenoy SG Evaluation of anti-inflammatory property of curcumin (diferuloyl methane) in patients with postoperative inflammation. International Journal of Clinical Pharmacology, Therapy, and Toxicology. 1986;**24**(12):651-654

[83] Ammon HP, Safayhi H, Mack T, Sabieraj J. Mechanism of antiinflammatory actions of curcumin and boswellic acids. Journal of Ethnopharmacology. 1993;**38**:113-119

[84] Jian YT, Wang JD, Mai GF, Zhang YL, Lai ZS. Curcumin regulates cyclooxygenase-2 activity in trinitrobenzene sulfonic acid-induced colitis. Journal of Fourth Military Medical University. 2005;**26**:521-524

[85] Skrzypczak-Jankun E, McCabe NP, Selman SH, Jankun J. Curcumin inhibits lipoxygenase by binding to its central cavity: Theoretical and X-ray evidence. International Journal of Molecular Medicine. 2000;**6**:521-526

[86] Joe B, et al. Presence of an acidic glycoprotein in the serum of arthritic rats: Modulation by capsaicin and curcumin. Molecular and Cellular Biochemistry. 1997;169(1-2):125-134

[87] Onodera S, Kaneda K, Mizue Y, Koyama Y, Fujinaga M, Nishihira J. Macrophage migration inhibitory factor up-regulates expression of matrix metalloproteinases in synovial fibroblasts of rheumatoid arthritis. The Journal of Biological Chemistry. 2000;**275**:444-450

[88] Lev-Ari S, Strier L, Kazanov D, Elkayam O, Lichtenberg D. Curcumin synergistically potentiates the growth-inhibitory and pro-apoptotic effects of celecoxib in osteoarthritis synovial adherent cells. Rheumatology (Oxford). 2006 Feb;**45**(2):171-7. Epub 2005 Oct 25

[89] Halpern GM. Anti-inflammatory effects of a stabilized lipid extract of Perna canaliculus (Lyprinol). Allergie und Immunologie. 2000;**32**:272-278

[90] Murphy KJ, Kiely M, Galvin K, Morrissey PA, Mann NJ, Sinclair AJ. New Zealand green lipped mussel (NZGLM) oil can reduce pro-inflammatory eicosanoids and cytokines and oxidation markers in vivo. Proceeding of the Nutrition Society of Australia. 2002;**26**:S289

[91] Brien S, Lewith G, Walker A, Hicks SM, Middleton D. Bromelain as a treatment for osteoarthritis: A review of clinical studies. Evidence-based Complementary and AlternativeMedicine. 2004;**1**:251-257

[92] Foster S, Tyler VE. Tyler's Honest Herbal: A Sensible Guide to the Use of Herbs and Related Remedies. Binghamton, NY: Haworth Herbal; 1999;39-41

[93] Totonchi A, Guyuron B. A randomized, controlled comparison between arnica and steroids in the management of postrhinoplasty ecchymosis and edema. Plastic and Reconstructive Surgery. 2007;**120**:271-274

[94] Karow JH, Abt HP, Frohling M, et al. Efficacy of arnica montana D4 for healing of wounds after Hallux valgus surgery compared to diclofenac. Journal of Alternative and Complementary Medicine. 2008;**14**:17-25

[95] Moore RA, Tramer MR, Carroll D, et al. Quantitative systematic review of topically applied non-steroidal anti-inflammatory drugs.BMJ. 1998;**316**:333-338

[96] Lyss G, Schmidt TJ, Merfort I, Pahl HL. Helenalin, an anti-inflammatory sesquiterpene lactone from Arnica, selectively inhibits transcription factor NF-kappaB. Biological Chemistry. 1997 Sep;**378**(9):951-61

[97] Schmidt C. A double-blind, placebo-controlled trial: Arnica montana applied topically to Subcutaneous mechanical injuries. Journal of the American Institute of Homeopathy. 1996;**89**:186

[98] Bellavite P. Historical background.Immunology and Homeopathy. 2005;**2**(4)441-452

[99] Frase W. La eficacia de las diluiciones homeopaticas en forma de acordes de potencias. Med Biol—Int J Biomed Res Ther. 1999;**12**(2):59-61

[100] Belon P, Cumps J, Ennis M, et al. Inhibition of human basophil degranulation by successive histamine dilutions: Results of a European multi-centre trial. Inflammation Research. 1999;**48**(suppl. 1):S17

[101] Belon P, Sainte-Laudy J. Inhibition of human basophil activation by high dilutions of histamine. Agents and Actions. 1993;**38**:C245-C247

[102] Carvalho AC, Bonamin LV. Efeito da administrac-a˜o de Arnica montana (tintura–ma˜e e preparac-o˜es dinamizadas 6CH) na atividade de diferentes agentes flogı´sticos em ratos. Pesq Hom. 2001;**16**:31-43

[103] Poitevin B, Aubin M, Royer JF. Belladonna and Ferrum phosphoricum effect in chemiluminiscence of polynuclear neutrophiles. Ann Hom Farina. 1983;**3**:5-12

[104] Winterberg H. Belladonna—Childhood diseases with particular reference to bronchitic inflammations. Biological Theroy of Journal Nature Medicine. 1986;**3**(4):79-81

[105] Galvaõ GG. A symptomatic totality's study of Stramonium, Belladonna and Hyoscyamus. Anais do XXI Congresso Brasileiro de Homeopatia.1992;**3**:35

[106] Bauer R. Echinacea drugs—effects and active ingredients. Zeitschrift fur Arztliche Fortbildung. 1996;**90**:111-115

[107] Wildfeuer A, Mayerhofer D. The effects of plant preparations on cellular functions in body defense. Arzeimttelforschung. 1994;**44**:361-366

[108] Hu C, Kitts DD. Studies on the antioxidant activity of Echinacea root extract. Journal of Agricultural and Food Chemistry. 2000;**48**:1466-1472

[109] Carvalho AC. Efeitos da administração de Arnica montana (tintura-mãe e UHD) na atividade de diferentes agentes flogísticos em ratos. In: Master of Science Dissertation. Instituto de Ciências da Saúde, Universidade Paulista—UNIP; Brasilia. 2000

[110] Macêdo SB, Ferreira LR, Perazzo FF, Tavares Carvalho JC. Anti-inflammatory activity of Arnica montana 6cH: Preclinical study in animals. Homeopathy. 2004;**93**:84-87

[111] Klaas CA, Wagner G, Laufer S et al.Studies on the anti-inflammatory activity of phytopharmaceuticals prepared from Arnica flowers. Planta Medica. 2002;**68**:385-391

[112] Bellavite P, Ortolani R, Conforti A.Immunology and homeopathy. Experimental studies on animal models. Evidence-based Complementary and Alternative Medicine. 2006;**3**:171-186

[113] Bellavite P, Conforti A, Pontarollo F, Ortolani R. Immunology and homeopathy. Cells of the immune system and inflammation. Evidence-Based Complementary and Alternative Medicine. 2006;**3**:13-24

[114] Conforti A, Bellavite P, Bertani S, Chiarotti F, Raschetti R. Rat models of acute inflammation: a randomized controlled study on the effects of homeopathic remedies. BMC Complementary and Alternative Medicine. 2007;**7**:1

[115] Palombo EA. Traditional medicinal plant extracts and natural products with activity against oral bacteria: Potential application in the prevention and treatment of oral diseases. Evidence-based Complementary and Alternative Medicine 2011;**2011**:680354

[116] Bonamin LV. Arnica montana and behavior of connective tissue. In: Signals and Images: Contributions and Contradictions of High Dilution Research. Springer; 2008. 113-125

[117] Fisher P, Scot DL. A randomized controlled trial of homeopathy in rheumatoid arthritis. Rheumatology. Oxford 2001;**40**:1052-1055

[118] Ballerini R, Casini A, Chinol M, Mannucci C, Giaccai L, Salvi M. Study on the absorption of ketoprofen topically administered in man: Comparison between tissue and plasma levels. International Journal of Clinical Pharmacology Research. 1986;**6**(1):69-72

[119] Dreiser RL. Topical antirheumatic drug therapy: Current practice and future trends. European Journal of Rheumatology and Inflammation. 1994;**14**(4):3-8. 27

[120] Brown MB, Martin GP, Jones SA, Akomeah FK. Dermal and transdermal drug delivery systems: Current and future prospects. Drug Delivery. 2006;**13**(3):175-187

[121] Fini A, Fazio G, Rapaport I. Diclofenac/N-(2-hydroxyethyl) pyrrolidine: A new salt for an old drug. Drugs under Experimental and Clinical Research. 1993;**19**(3):81-88

[122] Rusca A, Mautone G, Sun S, Magelli M, Johnson F. Comparison of plasma pharmacokinetics of FLECTOR® Patch (diclofenac epolaminetopical patch) and oral Voltaren® (diclofenac sodium enteric coated tablets) in healthy volunteers. The Journal of Pain. 2008;**9**(4 Suppl 1):45

[123] Zacher J, Altman RA, Bellamy N, et al. Topical diclofenac and its role in pain and inflammation: An evidence-based review. Current Medical Research and Opinion. 2008;**24**:925-950

[124] Barthel HR, Haselwood D, Longley S 3rd, Gold MS, Altman RD. Randomized controlled trial of diclofenac sodium gel in knee osteoarthritis. Seminars in Arthritis and Rheumatism. 2009 Dec;**39**(3):203-212

[125] Gallacchi G, Mautone G, Lualdi P. Painful inflammatory conditions: Topical treatment with diclofenac hydroxyethylpyrrolidine (Flector Gel 1%). Clinical Trials Journal. 1990;**27**(1):58-64

[126] Larkson PM, Haymes EM. Exercise and mineral status of athletes: Calcium, magnesium, phosphorus, and iron. Medicine and Science in Sports and Exercise. 1995;**27**:831-843

[127] Dickens BF, Weglicki WB, Li YS, Mak IT. Magnesium deficiency in vitro enhances free radical induced intracellular oxidative and cytotoxicity in endothelial cells. FEBS Letters. 1992;**311**:187-191

[128] Dominguez LJ, Barbagallo M, Lauretani F, Bandinelli S, et al. Magnesium and muscle performance in older persons: The InCHIANTI study. The American Journal of Clinical Nutrition. 2006;**84**:419-426

[129] Finstad EW, Newhouse IJ, Lukaski HC, McAuliffe JE, Stewart CR. The effects of magnesium supplementation on exercise performance. Medicine and Science in Sports and Exercise. 2001;**33**:493-498

[130] Volpe SL. Magnesium in disease prevention and overall health. Advances in Nutrition. 2013;**4**:378-383

[131] Watkins K, Josling PD. A Pilot Study to Determine the Impact of Transdermal Magnesium Treatment on Serum Levels and Whole Body CaMg Ratios. Spring; 2010

[132] Engen DJ, McAllister SJ, Whipple MO. Effects of transdermal magnesium chloride on quality of life for patients with fibromyalgia: A feasibility study. Journal of Integrative Medicine. 2015;**13**(5):306-313

[133] Barata F, Germano A , Di Lascio G. Establishment of galenic laboratories in developing countries to produce high quality medicines: results of Aid Progress Pharmacist Agreement (A.P.P.A.®) Project. Croatian Medical Journal. 2014;**55**(6):662-668

Chapter 6

Molecular Basis of Binding Interactions of NSAIDs and Computer-Aided Drug Design Approaches in the Pursuit of the Development of Cyclooxygenase-2 (COX-2) Selective Inhibitors

Pran Kishore Deb, Raghu Prasad Mailabaram,
Bilal Al-Jaidi and Mohamed Jamal Saadh

Additional information is available at the end of the chapter

http://dx.doi.org/10.5772/intechopen.68318

Abstract

The nonsteroidal anti-inflammatory drugs (NSAIDs) are important class of therapeutic agents used for the treatment of pain, inflammation and fever. Nonselective inhibition of cyclooxygenase (COX-1 and COX-2) isoenzymes by classical NSAIDs is associated with undesirable side effects such as gastrointestinal (GI) and renal toxicities due to COX-1 inhibition. To circumvent this problem, several COX-2 selective inhibitors were developed with superior GI safety profile. However, the voluntary market withdrawal of potent COX-2 selective inhibitors (rofecoxib and valdecoxib) due to their severe cardiovascular toxicity which is also found to be associated with some of the traditional NSAIDs suggesting the need to relook into the entire class of NSAIDs rather than exclusively victimizing the COX-2 selective inhibitors. Furthermore, the recent evidences for the involvement of COX-2 selective inhibitors in the aetiology of many diseases, such as Alzheimer's disease, Parkinson's disease, diabetes, various cancers and so on, have gained much attention for researchers to design and develop novel COX-2 selective inhibitors with improved pharmacodynamics and pharmacokinetic profile. This chapter is focused on the detailed analysis of molecular basis of binding interactions of various NSAIDs by highlighting the role of crucial amino acid residues at the binding site of cyclooxygenase enzymes (COXs) to be considered for selective inhibition of COX-2 enzyme while emphasising the impact of significant CADD strategies employed for designing new potent COX-2 inhibitors with tuned selectivity.

Keywords: molecular binding interactions of NSAIDs, computer-aided drug design of COX-2 selective inhibitors, development of COX-2 selective inhibitors

1. Introduction

The nonsteroidal anti-inflammatory drugs (NSAIDs) are important therapeutic agents used for the treatment of pain, inflammation and fever [1, 2]. NSAIDs act by reducing the production of pro-inflammatory prostaglandins (PGs) at the sites of injury through the obstruction of cyclooxygenase enzyme (COX) binding site by sterically preventing the binding of the endogenous arachidonic acid (AA) [1–3]. There are two different isoforms of COX isoenzymes, a constitutive form (COX-1) and an inducible form (COX-2), respectively [4]. The constitutive COX-1 isozyme plays an important role in many physiological functions, such as cytoprotection of gastric mucosa, renal blood flow regulation and platelet aggregation. The expression of COX-2 isozyme is mainly induced by several stimuli such as hormones, growth factors, mitogens, oncogenes and disorders of water-electrolyte homeostasis resulting in its involvement to pathological processes such as inflammation and various types of cancer [5]. The classical NSAIDs (aspirin, ibuprofen, flurbiprofen, naproxen, indomethacin, diclofenac, mefenamic acid, piroxicam, etc. (**Figure 1**)) are associated with side effects such as gastrointestinal (GI) ulcer and renal toxicity due to their nonselective inhibition of COX-1 pathway [6, 7]. As a result, a number of COX-2 selective inhibitors such as rofecoxib, celecoxib, valdecoxib and etoricoxib (**Figure 2**) were introduced into the market as safer NSAIDs which were devoid of GI toxicity. The voluntary market withdrawal of rofecoxib (Vioxx) by Merck in September 2004 based on APROVe (Adenomatous Polyp Prevention on Vioxx) study followed by valdecoxib (Bextra) in 2005 (Pfizer) due to their association with increased cardiovascular risk imposed a big question

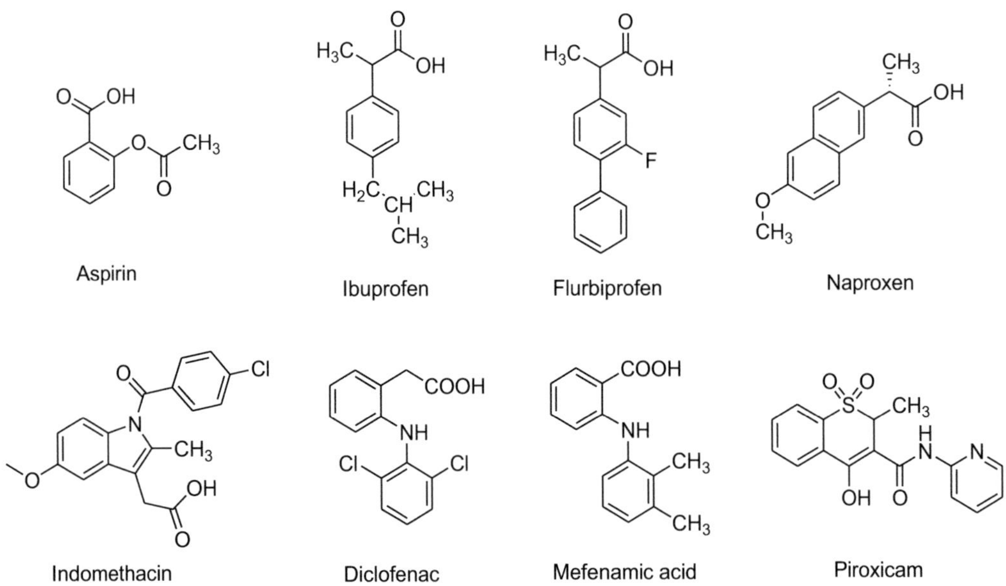

Figure 1. Representative structures of classical NSAIDs (nonselective COX inhibitors).

http://dx.doi.org/10.5772/intechopen.68318

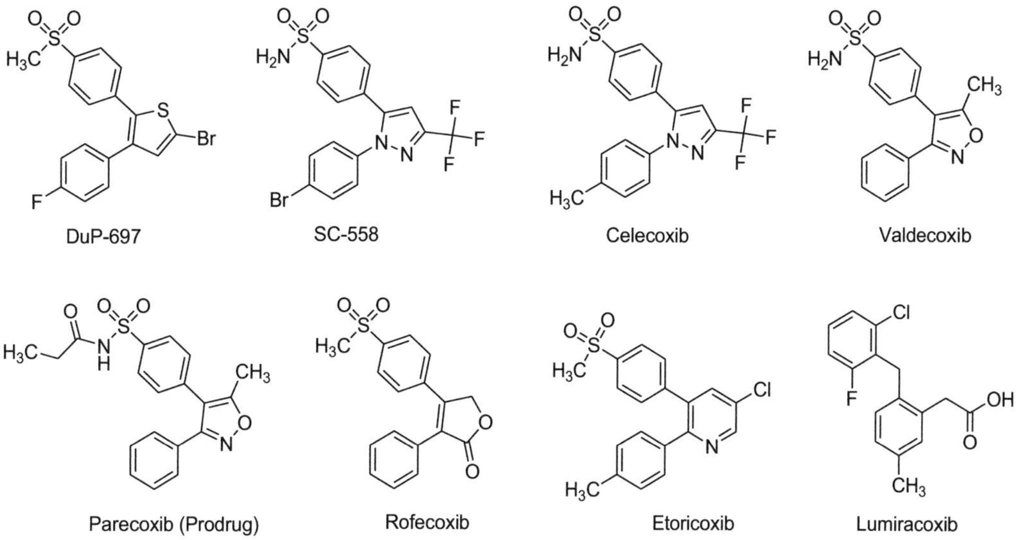

Figure 2. Structures of COX-2 selective inhibitors.

on the safety profile of this class of COX-2 selective inhibitors [8]. Interestingly, no such increased cardiovascular risk was observed from the Celecoxib Long-term Arthritis Safety Study (CLASS) trial. Celecoxib (Celebrex) is the only COX-2 selective inhibitor currently available in the US market with cautions of cardiac risk. Moreover, some of the nonselective NSAIDs such as high dosage of diclofenac and ibuprofen are also found to be associated with similar incidences of cardiovascular toxicity like COX-2 selective inhibitors [9]. Several research findings suggested that the adverse cardiovascular effects of COX-2 selective inhibitors might be dependent on the dose as well as duration of action [10–12]. However, the most potent COX-2 selective inhibitor, lumiracoxib (with different structures from other coxibs (**Figure 2**)), did not exhibit considerable cardiovascular adverse effects in Therapeutic Arthritis Research and Gastrointestinal Event Trial (TARGET) but found to be associated with serious hepatic toxicity which resulted in its withdrawal both from the Australian and European market [13, 14]. Furthermore, recent studies revealed the association of COX-2 with various other pathophysiological processes such as Alzheimer's disease, Parkinson disease, schizophrenia, epilepsy, depression, diabetic peripheral neuropathy and various cancers. [15, 16]. The recognition of new roles for COX-2 selective inhibitors imposed a great challenge to the researchers to design and explore alternative scaffolds to develop COX-2 selective inhibitors with improved potency and efficacy in order to circumvent various side effects associated with the currently available NSAIDs. Thus, a detailed analysis of the characteristic structural differences between the two isoenzymes along with the binding interactions of different NSAIDs is essential to construct a novel structure-based pharmacophore model for designing potent inhibitors with augmented COX-2 affinity as well as selectivity. This chapter is focused on the molecular basis of binding interactions of various NSAIDs by highlighting the role of crucial amino acid residues at the binding site of cyclooxygenase enzymes to be considered for selective inhibition of

COX-2 enzyme while emphasising the impact of various significant computer-aided drug design (CADD) approaches employed for designing new potent COX-2 inhibitors with tuned selectivity.

2. Progress in the pursuit of the development of cyclooxygenase-2 selective inhibitors

The discovery of the specific role of COX-2 enzyme in inflammation resulted in the development of several COX-2 selective inhibitors to overcome the GI side effects of classical NSAIDs [15, 16]. Interestingly, before the confirmation of existence of COX-2 enzyme, the DuPont company discovered a compound Dup-697 (**Figure 2**) as a potent anti-inflammatory agent without having the ulcerogenic effects of NSAIDs [17]. After the discovery of COX-2 enzyme, Dup-697 became the lead molecule for the development of COX-2 selective inhibitors (coxibs); as a result celecoxib and rofecoxib became the pioneer COX-2 selective inhibitors to reach the market [18, 19]. Dup-697 is a diaryl heterocyclic compound with cis-stilbene moiety. It has been observed from the structure-activity relationship (SAR) studies that the diaryl heterocyclic compounds possessing cis-stilbene moiety with variation in the para-position of one of the aryl rings play an important role in inducing selectivity for COX-2 as compared to COX-1 enzyme [20]. Celecoxib, valdecoxib and parecoxib (prodrug of valdecoxib) possess sulphonamide (SO_2NH_2) group, whereas etoricoxib and rofecoxib have a methyl sulphone (SO_2CH_3) group at the para-position of one of the aryl rings (**Figure 2**). Several attempts were made to extensively manipulate the ring system that is fused with the cis-stilbene system to include every possible heterocyclic ring of varying sizes as well as by altering the scaffolds of classical NSAIDs to convert them into COX-2 selective inhibitors, but none could successfully reach the market. Recently, a series of thiazole derivatives [21], cycloalkyl/aryl-3,4,5-trimethylgallates [22], thienopyrimidine derivatives [23], 3-alkoxy-4-methanesulfonamido acetophenone derivatives [24] and 8/10-trifluoromethyl-substituted-imidazo[1,2-*c*]quinazolines [25], have been designed, synthesised and reported from our research group in search of compounds with novel scaffold as potent anti-inflammatory agents.

Computer-aided drug design (CADD) strategies have been emerged as a potential tool for the discovery of new drugs. In the pursuit of the discovery and development of novel NSAIDs with selective inhibition of the COX-2 enzyme, various ligand-based 3D-QSAR and pharmacophore models were reported [15]. But these 3D-QSAR models are developed mainly based on particular classes of compounds which may not be applicable for the prediction of structurally diverse compounds. In contrast, the structure-based drug design approaches such as molecular docking and molecular dynamics (MD) simulation studies are based on detailed analysis of the binding site of target protein for designing novel drugs with improved potency. The availability of various 3D X-ray crystal structures of COX-1 and COX-2 isoenzymes co-crystallised with diverse selective and nonselective inhibitors provides an opportunity to gain insight into various physicochemical requirements for effective binding of a ligand with selective inhibition of COX-2.

3. Structural and functional insights of cyclooxygenase enzymes

The COX-1 enzyme is constitutively expressed in most tissues where it is encoded by PTGS-1 gene (codes for a relatively stable 2.8 kb mRNA). On the other hand, COX-2 is encoded by PTGS-2 gene (codes for a relatively less stable 4 kb mRNA), which is activated by several inflammatory and proliferative stimuli [3]. The difference in gene expression account for the existence of two COX isoforms, signifying that COX-1 provides PGs essential for maintaining homeostasis including gastric cytoprotection, whereas COX-2 plays an important role in producing PGs during various pathological conditions such as inflammation and tumourigenesis [26]. These observations became the driving force for the rapid development of COX-2 selective inhibitors having anti-inflammatory activity while avoiding GI side effects associated with traditional nonselective NSAIDs.

Human COX-1 and COX-2 enzymes exist as homodimers of 576 and 581 amino acids, respectively, and each monomer having a molecular mass of about 70 kDa [3, 26]. Both enzymes are almost identical in their general tertiary structure with 60% sequence similarity. The signal peptide of COX-1 is longer (with seven amino acid residues) than COX-2, and the N-terminus of COX-1 has an insertion of eight residues, while the C-terminus of COX-2 has an insertion of eighteen residues. Each subunit of COX-1 and COX-2 dimers consists of three structural domains: the N-terminal epidermal growth factor (EGF) domain (amino acid residues 34–72), the α-helical membrane-binding domain (amino acid residues 73–116) and the C-terminal catalytic domain, which comprises the bulk of the protein. The catalytic domain contains the cyclooxygenase and peroxidase active sites on either side of the heme prosthetic group [26–28]. Recent studies revealed that only one monomer of the COX homodimer is active at a given time [29]. It has been postulated that these monomers can act additionally through an allosteric/catalytic couple, with AA oxygenation being controlled in the 'catalytic' monomer (E_{cat}) through the binding of non-substrate fatty acids and nonselective NSAIDs to the opposite monomer, the 'allosteric' monomer (E_{allo}) [30, 31]. Moreover, the major differences between COX-1 and COX-2 are the substitutions of the bulkier amino acid residues Ile434, His513 and Ile523 in COX-1 by comparatively smaller residues Val434, Arg513 and Val523, respectively, in COX-2 at the main channel of cyclooxygenase binding site (**Figure 3**). These substitutions produce a 25% increase in the volume of the active site at COX-2 along with

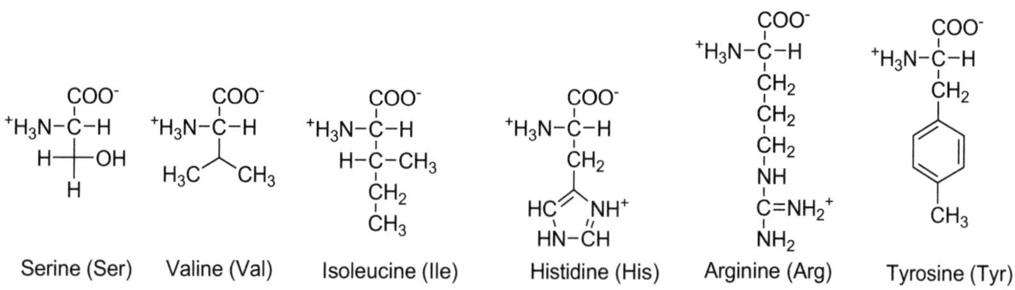

Figure 3. Structures of amino acid residues playing crucial role at the active site of COX enzymes.

the creation of a side pocket off the main channel with Arg513 located at its base [26]. The sulphonamide or methyl sulphone moieties of diaryl heterocycle-based coxibs were mainly designed to bind within this side pocket to provide selective inhibition of COX-2.

4. Molecular basis of inhibition of cyclooxygenase enzymes and computer-aided drug design (CADD) approaches employed for the design and discovery of COX-2 selective inhibitors

The experimental methodologies such as site-directed mutagenesis, X-ray crystallographic analysis along with various CADD approaches such as structure-based molecular docking studies (employing Amber, Flexi dock, Fast dock, Glide), MD simulation, metadynamics simulation studies and ligand-based 3D-QSAR (by using COMFA, COMSiA) and pharmacophore modelling were extensively used to understand the molecular basis of interactions of NSAIDs with COX enzymes as well as to design novel potent COX-2 selective inhibitors. The site-directed mutagenesis and X-ray crystallographic structures of COX-1 and COX-2 isoenzymes indicate that selective and nonselective inhibitors generally bind in two different patterns which provides an impetus for the rational modulation of existing binders to improve selectivity and potency. It has been observed that the selectivity pocket of COX-1 is comparatively smaller due to the presence of bulky amino acid residue Ile523, whereas in COX-2 the presence of smaller amino acid residue Val523 enlarged the selectivity pocket providing a more stable binding opportunity for selective inhibitors [32, 33]. Further, the kinetics of selective and nonselective inhibitors were found to be different, and it has been postulated that the association of COX-2 selective inhibitor SC-299 with COX-1 and COX-2 occurs at similar rate, while the dissociation of SC-299 from COX-2 is 100-fold slower than COX-1 indicating the correlation between the relative rate of dissociation and the selective inhibition of COX-2 isoenzyme [34]. This correlation was also confirmed by Walker et al. in additional experiments on other COX-2 selective inhibitors [35]. The stable binding mode of selective inhibitors to COX-2 isoform is also attributed to the presence of a different amino acid residue Val434 instead of Ile434 as found in the binding site of COX-1 enzyme.

The active site of COX-2 is mainly hydrophobic where most of the protein-ligand interactions are stabilised by van der Waals forces. According to the X-ray crystal structure of COX-2 bound with the SC-558 (PDB: 1CX2; 2.5 Å resolution) [33], the ligand binds in the cyclooxygenase active site where the bromophenyl ring occupies a hydrophobic pocket formed by Tyr348, Phe381, Leu384, Tyr385, Trp387, Gly526, Ala527 and Ser530, respectively (**Figure 4**). The trifluoromethyl group attached to the pyrazole ring is surrounded by a close hydrophobic cavity formed by Met113, Val116, Val349, Tyr355, Leu359 and Leu531 where only Arg120 (located near to CF_3 group) introduces a strong electrostatic field. This cavity is referred to as common pocket (**Figure 4A**) as it is also found to be occupied by the aromatic ring bearing the carboxylate functional group of many nonselective COX inhibitors such as ibuprofen and flurbiprofen, respectively [38]. Furthermore, these two features of SC-558 binding are almost equivalent to the binding mode of flurbiprofen and indomethacin [33]. The phenylsulphonamide moiety of

(A)

(B)

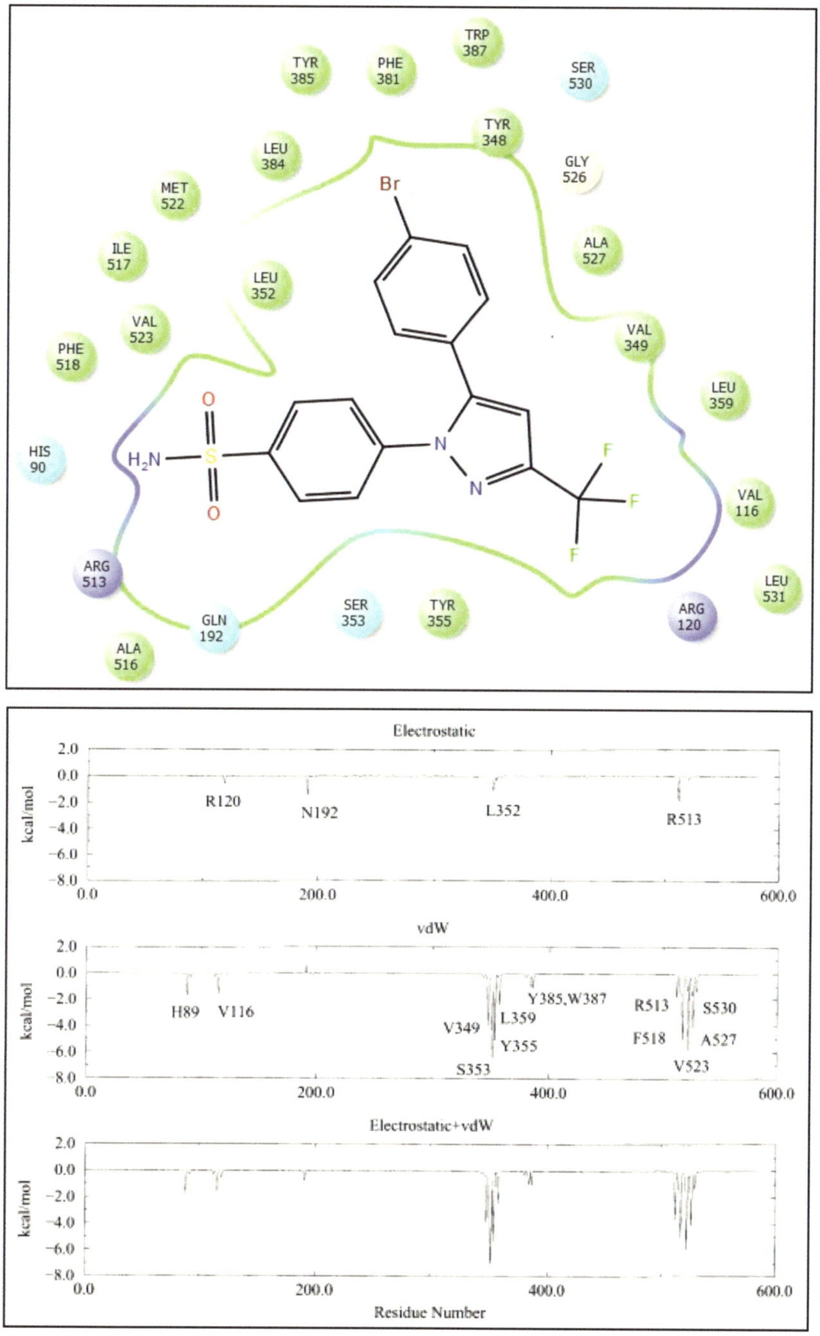

Figure 4. (A) 2D X-ray crystallographic pose of SC-558 in COX-2 (unpublished pose taken with the help maestro academic visualiser 10.4 [36] by using the crystal structure of COX-2, PDB ID: 1CX2). (B) UBEXTRACT plots (electrostatic, van der Waals and total energy) for the interaction of SC-558 with the different residues of the protein (values shown correspond to the average of 1.5 ns of MD simulation) (reprinted with permission from Robert et al. [37], copyright © 2003 American Chemical Society).

SC-558 is found to be anchored within a selectivity pocket formed by His90, Asn192, Leu352, Ser353, Arg513, Ala516, Ile517, Phe518 and Val523 assuming a conformation in which one of the oxygen atoms forms H-bond with Arg513 and is close enough to interact with His90, while the amide hydrogens are able to interact with the backbone of Phe518 through two water bridges. The phenylsulphonamide moiety of SC-558 is mainly responsible for inducing selectivity for COX-2, where it is easily accessible to the selectivity pocket due to the presence of smaller residue Val523 that is more restricted in COX-1 because of the substitution of valine to isoleucine at the same position-523 [33, 38].

Robert et al. demonstrated the binding mechanism of different NSAIDs (mainly celecoxib and rofecoxib analogues) to the cyclooxygenase active site of COX-2 based on molecular dynamics (MD) simulation and free energy calculation studies [37]. The MD simulation study carried out by using the homology model of human COX-2 also revealed similar binding mode of interaction of SC-558 as observed from crystallographic pose [33]. To investigate the key residues involved in the interaction of NSAIDs with COX-2, the MD trajectories were analysed by using UBEXTRACT programme. For example, the UBEXTRACT analysis [37] indicated that mainly four residues (Arg120, Asn192, Leu352 and Arg513) made significant electrostatic interactions, whereas thirteen residues involved in van der Waals interaction with the SC-558 (**Figure 4B**). The inspection of experimental data of valdecoxib suggested that the methyl group attached to the central isoxazole ring is favourable for binding by making hydrophobic interaction. The MD simulation study of rofecoxib [37] showed that the carbonyl group of furanone ring formed an H-bond with Ser530. It is interesting to note that to achieve this contact the side chain of Ser530 adopted a 'down orientation', whereas it favours 'up conformation' while interacting with celecoxib because of water-mediated H-bond between Ser530 and Tyr385 residues (**Figure 5A** and **B**).

Vittorio et al. used an advanced metadynamics-based computational technique to simulate the full dissociation process of a highly potent and selective inhibitor SC-558 in both COX-1 and COX-2 isoenzymes [38]. The metadynamics study of SC-558 dissociation process in COX-2 was able to reproduce the X-ray crystallographic pose and also revealed the possibility of an alternative binding mode (**Figure 6A** and **B**). In this alternative binding mode (**Figure 6B**), the bromophenyl moiety is found to be anchored within a highly hydrophobic cavity formed by Ile345, Val349, Leu359, Leu531 and Met535, while the trifluoromethylpyrazole moiety undergone 180° rotation which resulted in improved interactions with neighbouring residues such as Leu352, Phe518, Val523, Gly526 and Ala527, respectively. Finally, the sulphonamide group engages in the formation of H-bond with Tyr355 and Arg120 (**Figure 6B**). Similar observation is also evident from another study where the mutation Tyr355Phe disfavoured the binding of many ligands to COX [40]. Further support to this alternative binding mode of SC-558 comes from the very similar binding mode of some of the experimentally observed nonselective COX inhibitors, in particular the binding mode of ibuprofen to COX-1 (PDB ID: 1EQG) where the main interactions with the protein are well conserved [41]. The carboxylate group of ibuprofen forms polar interactions with Tyr355 and Arg120 similarly to the sulphonamide moiety of SC-558 (**Figure 6C**). In either case, the common pocket is occupied by the phenyl ring in ibuprofen and the pyrazole moiety in SC-558. The similarity is even greater in case of flurbiprofen or diclofenac, where a halogen atom is substituted in the phenyl ring enforcing the hydrophobic interactions with Leu352, Phe518 and Val523 similar to trifluoromethyl group of SC-558 (in alternative pose).

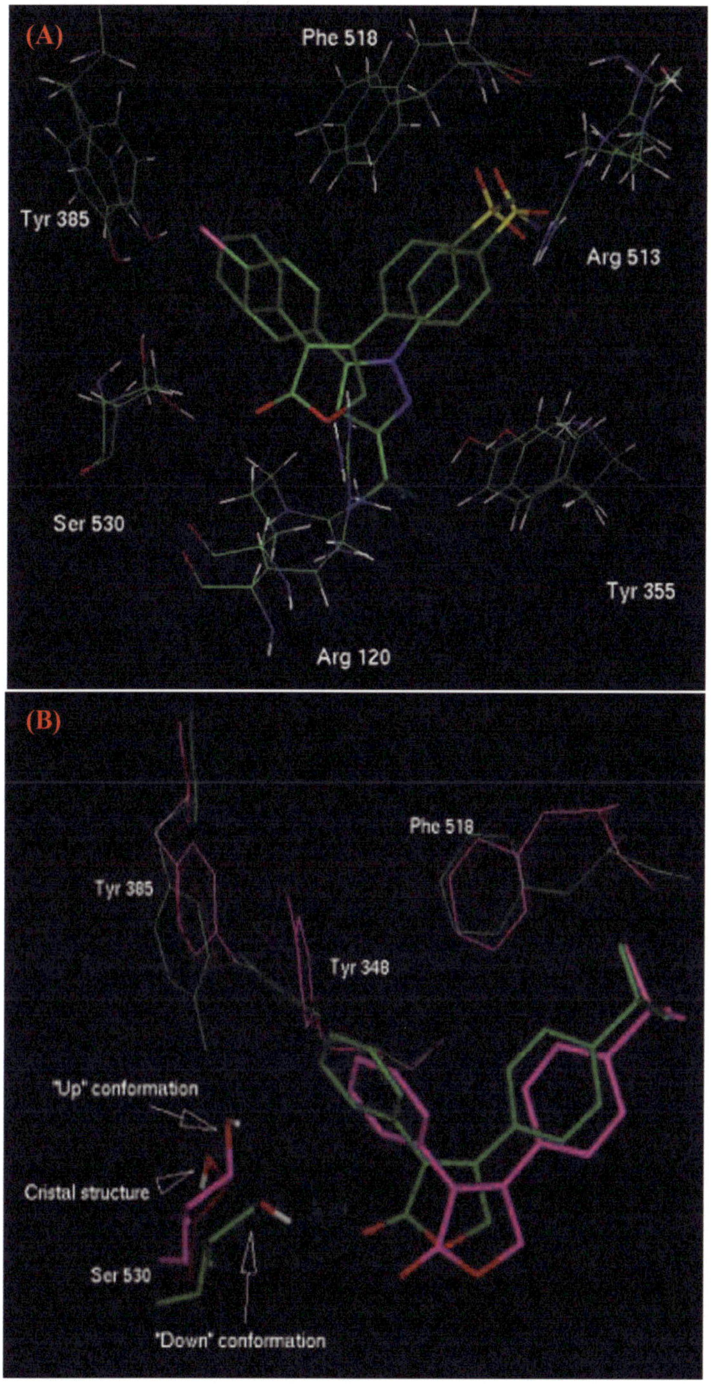

Figure 5. (A) Comparison of the SC-558 and rofecoxib binding modes after superposition of both protein binding sites. (B) Details of the rofecoxib binding site when Ser530 is in the 'up' (magenta) and in the 'down' (green) conformation. The conformation found in the crystal structure (brown) is also displayed for comparison (reprinted with permission from Robert et al. [37], copyright © 2003 American Chemical Society).

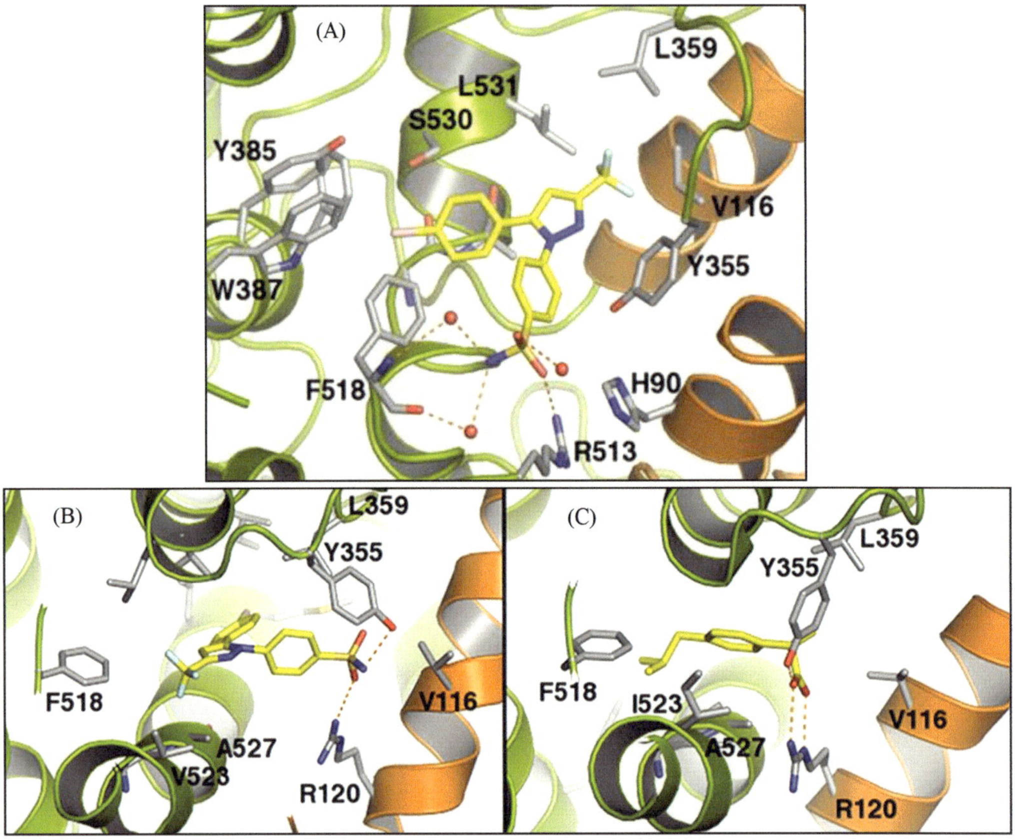

Figure 6. (A) The X-ray crystallographic pose of SC-558 in COX-2 (PDB ID code 1CX2) reproduced during the metadynamics simulations. (B) The alternative binding pose of SC-558 in COX-2 found during metadynamics simulations. (C) The X-ray binding conformation of ibuprofen in complex with COX-1 (PDB ID code 1EQG). The ligands are represented as yellow, whereas the protein is represented as green cartoon with the α-helices forming the gate coloured in orange and the hydrogens are not displayed for clarity (reprinted with permission from Vittorio et al. [38]).

The experimentally observed time-dependent slow tight-binding inhibition of other diaryl heterocyclic compounds similar to SC-558 is interpreted due to the presence of an additional binding step, where a vital role might be played by the rearrangement of the hydrogen-bonding network formed by Arg120, Tyr355 and Glu524, respectively, which are assumed to be critical for the transition from the relaxed to the tightened state of the enzyme. The involvement of these key residues (Arg120 and Tyr355) in the newly observed alternative binding mode of SC-558 suggests that the time-dependent inhibition kinetics of SC-558 results from the ability of the ligand to bind in two distinct but equally strong ways [38].

The metadynamics simulation study of SC-558 dissociation process in COX-1 reveals that the conformation of SC-558 in COX-1 is very similar to the crystallographic pose of SC-558 in COX-2, where the ligand is more weakly bound because of the partial insertion of the sulphonamide group into the selectivity pocket of COX-1 due to the presence of bulkier Ile523 in contrast to Val523 in COX-2 [38]. Moreover, the presence of the bulkier residue Ile523 in COX-1

http://dx.doi.org/10.5772/intechopen.68318

also nullifies the occurrence of alternative binding mode that is observed in case of COX-2 binding interaction. This hypothesis of selective inhibitors with their high residence time in COX-2 due to the existence of additional binding step/mode is also evident from another study on a series of COX-2 selective inhibitors [34, 35]. The binding conformation of SC-558 in COX-1 determined through metadynamics simulation study is very similar to the crystallographic pose found for celecoxib in COX-1 [39] with a low RMSD of 1.46 Å for the ligand heavy atoms.

The analysis of X-ray crystallographic binding mode of Vioxx (rofecoxib) with huCOX-2 (PDB ID: 5KIR) [42] shows that the inhibitor makes a total of 42 contacts with amino acid residues (mainly hydrophobic in nature), while the methyl sulphone moiety occupies the side pocket of the cyclooxygenase channel and the phenyl ring extended up towards the side chain of Tyr385 (**Figure 7A–C**). The oxygen (O) atoms of the methyl sulphone moiety of the inhibitor

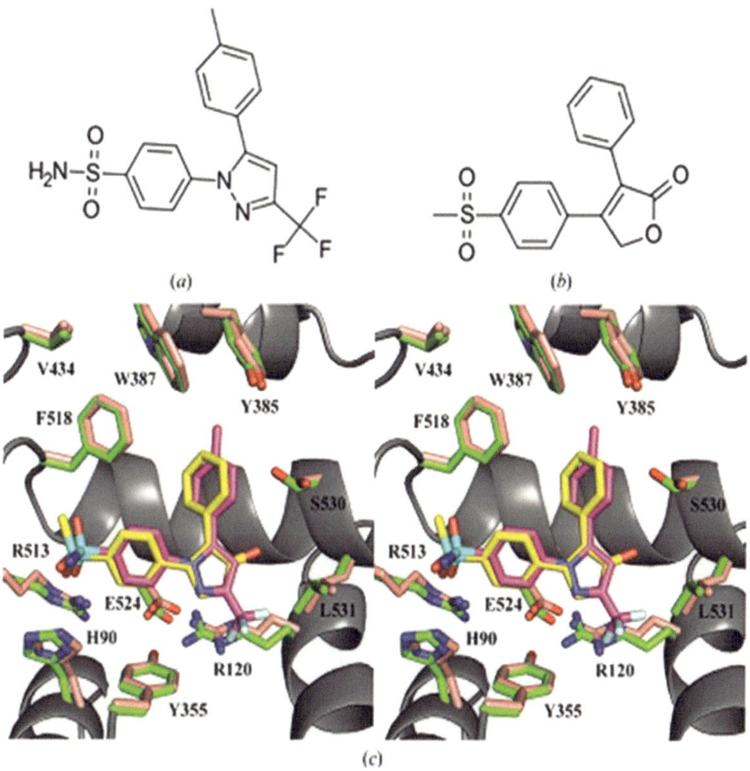

Figure 7. Comparison of celecoxib and Vioxx (rofecoxib) bound within the cyclooxygenase channel of COX-2. (A and B) Chemical structures of (A) celecoxib and (B) Vioxx. Although both inhibitors share a common diaryl heterocycle scaffold, celecoxib contains a pyrazole heterocycle and a sulphonamide moiety, whereas Vioxx contains a furanone heterocycle and a methyl sulphone moiety. (C) Stereoview showing an overlay of Vioxx (yellow) and celecoxib (magenta) from PDB entry 3LN1 bound within the cyclooxygenase channel of COX-2 (C^{α} r.m.s.d. of 0.31 A° for 542 pairs). The binding mode of the two coxibs is conserved, with the sulphone/sulphonamide moieties penetrating into the COX-2-specific side pocket. C-atoms of residues lining the channel are coloured green for huCOX-2 and salmon for muCOX-2, whereas N- and O-atoms are coloured blue and red, respectively (reprinted with permission from Orlando and Malkowski [42]).

made the only significant hydrophilic interactions with the side-chain N-atoms of His90 and Arg513, respectively, positioned at the base of the side pocket. It is surprising to note that Vioxx is approximately 60-fold more COX-2 selective than celecoxib [43], but it binds in the same general conformation as evident from celecoxib binding within the cyclooxygenase active site (**Figure 7C**) [44]. The reason for the difference in COX-2 selectivity between these two inhibitors presumed to be because of their differences in binding kinetics rather than in a particular enzyme-inhibitor interaction. Hence, the binding and dissociation kinetic analysis of both Vioxx and celecoxib might provide a clear rationale for their different degrees of isoform selectivity.

Further, the X-ray crystallographic pose of celecoxib/ovCOX-1 [39] shows that the Ile523 propagates a shift of side-chain residues such as His513, Pro514 and Asn515 in the β-turn loop of the 'side pocket' (**Figure 8**). The trifluoromethyl (CF_3) group attached to the pyrazole ring of celecoxib does not interact with Arg120 typically observed with substrates and other carboxylic acid-containing inhibitors. Instead, the trifluoromethyl group adjoins Tyr355 where the phenyl ring of Tyr355 makes edge-to-face contact with the aromatic ring of the benzene-sulphonamide group of celecoxib (**Figure 8**). It has been also observed that both inhibitors, SC-558 and celecoxib, bind in a similar manner with two exceptions. The sulphonamide group forms a hydrogen bond with His513 in ovCOX-1 which is Arg513 in muCOX-2. In ovCOX-1, the rigid histidine residue does not form a hydrogen bond with celecoxib. The amide nitrogen of sulphonamide moiety of celecoxib forms short N—H—O H-bonds with the side chain of Gln192 and main chain of Leu352 (**Figure 8**). Moreover, Ile434 (Val434 in COX-2) is proposed to act as a gate to prevent Phe518 from moving away when bound to COX-2 selective inhibitors. As a result, Phe518 forms hydrophobic contacts with the benzene ring of the inhibitor in COX-1.

The most commonly used nonselective NSAID, aspirin, covalently modifies COX-1 and COX-2 in a time-dependent manner via the acetylation of the hydroxyl group of Ser-530 [45].

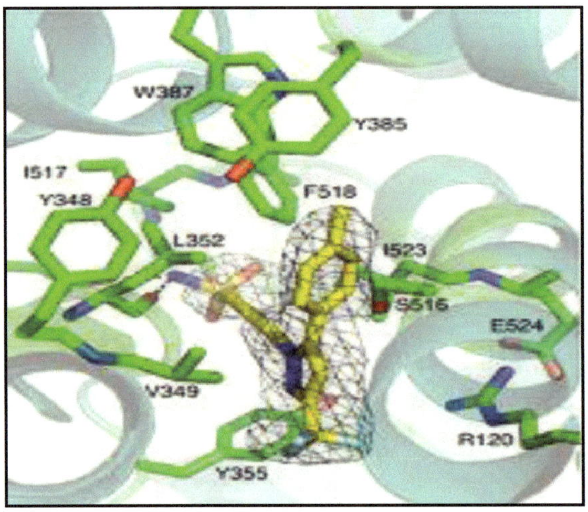

Figure 8. Celecoxib binding to ovCOX-1 as determined by X-ray crystallography [39] (reprinted with permission from Gilad et al. [39]).

The binding mode of flurbiprofen is found to be identical in both COX-1 and COX-2 (PDB ID: 3PGH) isoenzymes [33]. Moreover, it also shows similarity with the binding mode of two features of SC-558, where the distal phenyl ring and the fluorophenyl ring of flurbiprofen superimpose with the bromophenyl ring and pyrazole ring of SC-558, respectively. In contrast, the distal phenyl ring of flurbiprofen forms a π-stacking interaction with Tyr385 while interacting with Ser530, the residue that is selectively acetylated by aspirin, whereas the carboxylate group forms a salt bridge with the guanidine moiety of Arg120 and a hydrogen bond with Tyr355, respectively (**Figure 9B**). Furthermore, the fluorine atom of fluorophenyl ring interacts with the side chain of Ile523 in COX-1, which is absent in COX-2 because of the presence of a smaller residue valine at the corresponding position-523.

Similarly, the X-ray crystallographic binding mode of another nonselective COX inhibitor, indomethacin (PDB ID: 4COX) [33], reveals that it anchors well within the cyclooxygenase active site of COX-2 (**Figure 9A**) by forming a salt bridge between the carboxylate group and guanidine moiety of Arg120 (similar to flurbiprofen), while the indole ring mainly interacts with Val349 and Ser353 and forms additional contact with Tyr355, Val523 and Ala527, respectively. The six-member ring of indole forms close interaction with Leu352 and Ser353, whereas the *o*-methoxy group protrudes slightly into a relatively large cavity adjacent to Ser353, Tyr355 and Val523 in COX-2. The benzoyl group occupies a position very similar to that of the distal phenyl ring of flurbiprofen and forms stable hydrophobic interactions with Phe381, Leu384, Tyr385 and Trp387, respectively, while the benzoyl oxygen forms H-bonding interactions with side-chain hydroxyl group of Ser530 and with Val349, and the chlorine atom interacts with Leu384. It has to be noted that the benzoyl ring can adopt either *cis* or *trans* conformation with respect to indole ring and possibility of *cis* conformation is claimed to be preferable based on the conformation of indomethacin complex with COX-1. It has also been anticipated that the benzoyl oxygen plays a vital role in enhancing the affinity for COX-1.

Duggan et al. in their study based on site-directed mutagenesis and X-ray crystallography, postulated that the binding mode of naproxen (**Figure 9C**) is similar to other members of the 2-arylpropionic acid family of NSAIDs [46]. It is important to note that the majority of 2-arylpropionic acid family of NSAIDs are marketed as racemic mixtures except naproxen which is exclusively sold as the (*S*)-enantiomer. The (*S*)-α-methyl group of naproxen plays a crucial role by forming a critical interaction with the COX enzymes and occupies into a hydrophobic cleft below Val-349, whereas the removal or substitution of methyl group with a range of substituents of varying size and stereochemistry at the α-position results in a dramatic loss of potency. The carboxylate group makes hydrogen-bonding interactions with Arg-120 and Tyr-355 at the base of the active site. The *p*-methoxy group of naproxen forms van der Waals interactions with Tyr-385 and Trp-387, while the naphthyl moiety of naproxen makes hydrophobic interactions with Ala-527, Gly-526 and Leu-352, respectively (**Figure 9C**). It has been observed that the side chain of Leu-352 adopts an alternate conformation as compared to that observed in case of binding interactions of co-crystal structures of flurbiprofen, indomethacin and diclofenac bound to mCOX-2 (**Figure 9A–D**) [46].

Comparative analysis of X-ray crystal structures of other 2-arylpropionic acids and the diaryl heterocyclic compounds bound to the COX enzymes shows that the α-methyl or

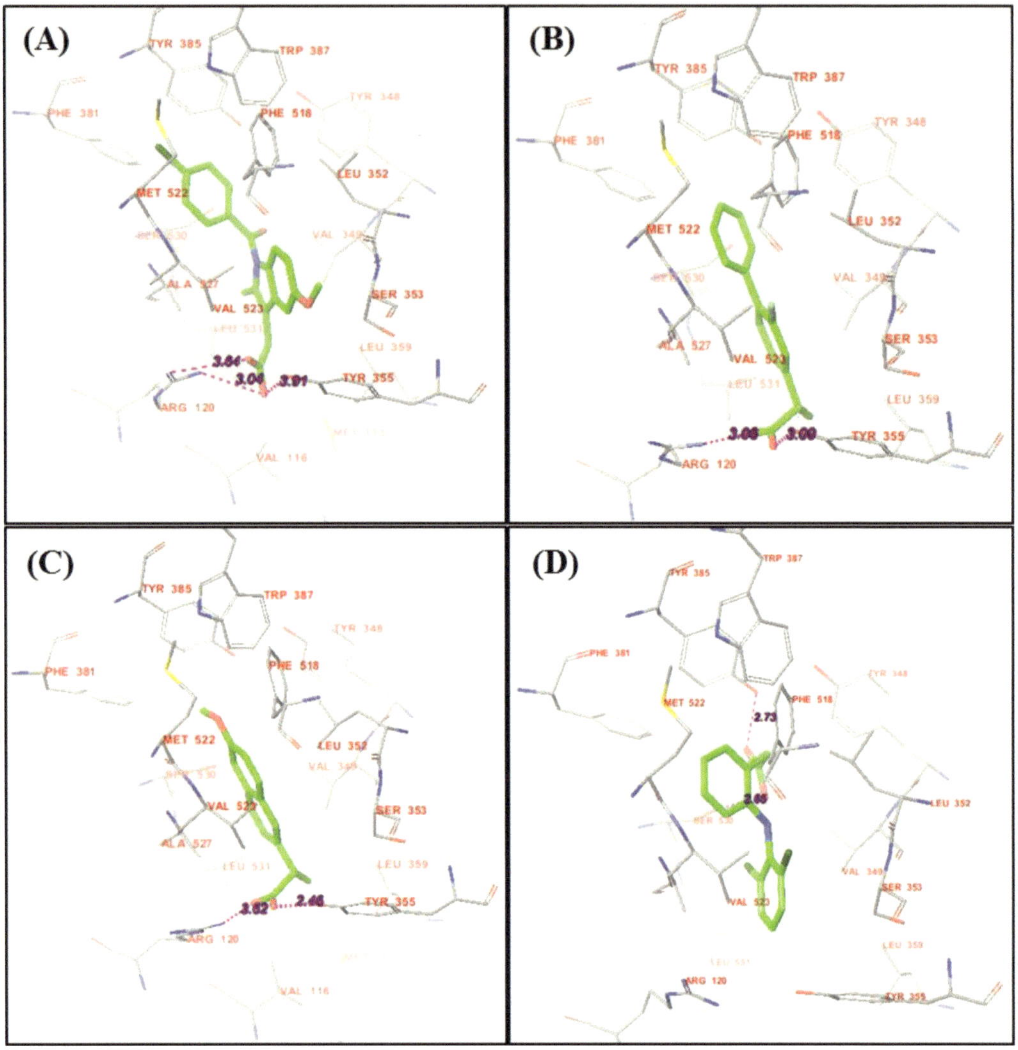

Figure 9. (A) Binding mode of the crystal structure of indomethacin (PDB ID: 4COX) at the COX-2 active site showing H-bonding with constriction residues Arg-120 and Tyr-355 at the base of the active site. (B) Binding mode of the crystal structure of flurbiprofen (PDB ID: 3PGH) at the COX-2 active site showing H-bonding with constriction residues Arg-120 and Tyr-355. (C) Binding mode of the crystal structure of naproxen (PDB ID: 3NT1) at the COX-2 active site showing H-bonding with constriction residues Arg-120 and Tyr-355 (similar to indomethacin and flurbiprofen). The inhibitor does not enter the side pocket into which the phenyl sulphonamide or phenyl sulphone moieties of diaryl heterocyclic compounds protrude. (D) Binding mode of the crystal structure of diclofenac (PDB ID: 1PXX) bound at the COX-2 active site showing the opposing binding mode where the position of acidic groups coordinated to the catalytic Tyr-385 as well as Ser-530 at the top of the pocket. The inhibitor carbon atoms are coloured green. All the poses were taken with the help of maestro academic visualiser 10.4, Schrodinger [36].

4-trifluoromethyl (SC-558) group makes interaction in a similar manner to the naproxen [33, 41]. Interestingly, COX inhibitors belonging to carboxylate-containing family without having a methyl group in the α-position exploit different interactions to reinforce binding within the active site of COX enzymes. For example, diclofenac binds with an inverted orientation (**Figure 9D**) where the carboxylate group makes H-bonds with Ser-530 and Tyr-385 and a chlorine atom attached to the lower aniline ring occupies into a hydrophobic pocket above Val-349.

Juan et al. carried out docking studies by using the AMBER programme to provide proper insights of the differential binding mode of diverse families of COX inhibitors, including selective and nonselective ligands: rofecoxib, ketoprofen, suprofen, carprofen, zomepirac, indomethacin, diclofenac and meclofenamic, respectively [47]. Their study concluded the importance of several structural features that should be attached to a scaffold required for efficient COX inhibition such as (i) a carboxylate moiety essential for interaction with the Arg120 side chain, (ii) a carbonyl moiety important for making hydrogen bond with the side chain of Ser530 and (iii) a distal aromatic ring crucial for fitting into a hydrophobic pocket underneath the Tyr385 side chain. Desiraju et al. reported 3D-QSAR models with high predictive abilities from a set of 114 substituted 1,2-diarylimidazole analogues for computer-aided design of COX-2 selective inhibitors based on 3D-QSAR studies employing comparative molecular field analysis (CoMFA) and comparative molecular similarity indices analysis (CoMSIA) approaches, by including hydrophobic (lipophilic), electrostatic, steric and hydrogen bond donor and acceptor fields as well as docking studies with FlexiDock (using the X-ray crystal structures of COX-1 and COX-2 with PDB ID: 1PGG and 6COX, respectively) [48]. Adinarayana et al. studied the interactions of COX-2 active site residues with selective inhibitors (rofecoxib, etoricoxib, valdecoxib, celecoxib and its analogues) and assessed the importance of scoring functions based on docking studies employing X-score scoring function and FastDock programme. The study concluded that the main interactions of COX-2 inhibitors within the binding pocket enzymes are hydrogen bonding and hydrophobic interactions indicating that sulphonamide and substituted pyrazole groups act as potential pharmacophore features for the design of highly potent and COX-2 selective inhibitors [49]. Sundar et al. developed a virtual library of drug-like novel molecules by employing structure-based de novo drug designing and 2D-fingerprinting approaches followed by molecular docking and MD simulation studies and reported two compounds as promising highly COX-2 selective inhibitors [50]. Chakraborti et al. in their extensive review [15] highlighted various molecular modelling-based approaches in search of novel potential COX-2 selective inhibitors overcoming various side effects posed by the drugs in clinical use.

Recently, Pfizer Global Research and Development, USA [51], reported their structure-based drug design efforts and discovery of two novel orally available benzopyran class of COX-2 selective inhibitors (SD-8381 and SC-75416, structurally different from the diaryl heterocycle class of coxibs (**Figure 10**)) under clinical trials with superior potency and efficacy as an anti-inflammatory and analgesic agent as compared to other NSAIDs and COX-2 selective inhibitors. In particular, the compound SC-75416 exhibited a human half-life of 34 h, which is suitable for once daily dosing and also demonstrated superior analgesic efficacy in a phase II clinical trial of postsurgical dental pain. However, the entire membrane-binding helix cluster and the side chain of Tyr355 observed to move ~0.7 and 1.6 Å away from the active site to accommodate the bulky 7-*t*-butyl substituent. The binding orientation of both the compounds is very similar to each other and conserves many similar contacts between the

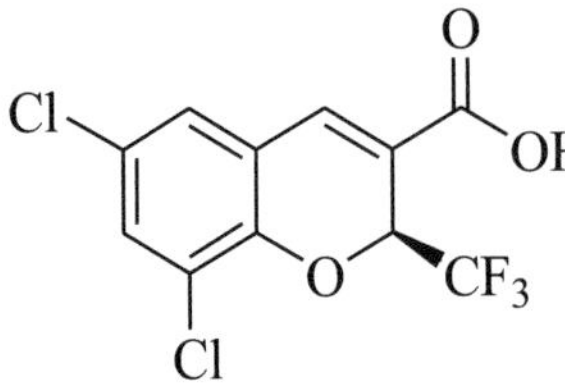

SD-8381

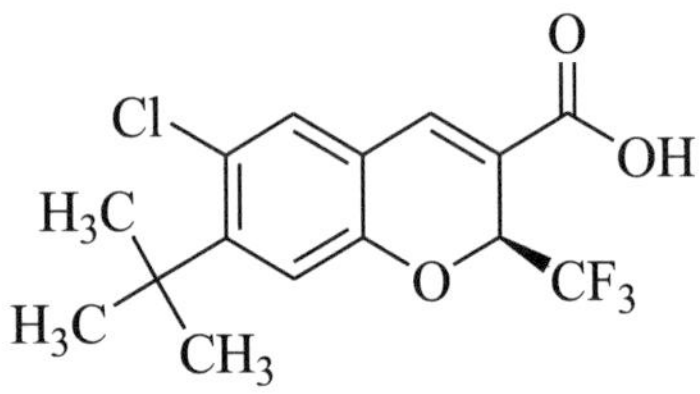

SC-75416

Figure 10. Chemical structures and biological data of novel benzopyran derivatives SD-8381 and SC-75416 [51].

enzyme and inhibitor, while the carboxylate group makes H-bond interactions with Tyr385 and Ser530, respectively.

5. Conclusion

Traditional NSAIDs act by nonselective inhibition of cyclooxygenase isoenzymes and are found to be associated with various undesirable side effects such as gastrointestinal (GI) and renal toxicity due to COX-1 inhibition. As a result, a number of COX-2 selective inhibitors (celecoxib, rofecoxib, valdecoxib, etc.) were developed as safer NSAIDs with improved GI safety profile. But the voluntary market withdrawal of rofecoxib and valdecoxib due to their strong association with cardiovascular toxicity imposed a big question on the safety profile of COX-2 selective inhibitors. However, similar cardiovascular toxicity was also found to be associated with some of the traditional NSAIDs suggesting the need to relook into the entire class of NSAIDs rather than exclusively victimising the COX-2 selective inhibitors. Furthermore, the recent evidences for the involvement of COX-2 selective inhibitors in the aetiology of many diseases, such as Alzheimer's disease, Parkinson's disease, diabetes, various cancers, etc. have gained much attention of researchers to design and develop novel COX-2 selective inhibitors with improved pharmacodynamic and pharmacokinetic profile. The availability of 3D X-ray crystal structures of cyclooxygenase enzymes (COX-1 and COX-2) co-crystallised with diverse selective as well as nonselective inhibitors provides an opportunity to gain insight into various physicochemical requirements of ligands for effective binding with selective inhibition of COX-2 enzyme. The main differences between COX-1 and COX-2 are found to be the substitutions of the bulkier amino acid residues Ile434, His513 and Ile523 in COX-1 by comparatively smaller residues Val434, Arg513 and Val523, respectively, in COX-2 at the main channel of cyclooxygenase binding site which resulted in the 25% increase in the volume of the active site at COX-2. The advancement of CADD approaches made a great impact in the discovery process by facilitating the proper understanding of the differential molecular interactions of various inhibitors with cyclooxygenase enzymes. The detailed analysis of molecular basis of binding interactions of NSAIDs and various insightful CADD approaches discussed in this chapter will be useful to build new strategies to develop novel potential COX-2 selective inhibitors to circumvent the limitations associated with the NSAIDs in clinical use.

Author details

Pran Kishore Deb[1]*, Raghu Prasad Mailabaram[2], Bilal Al-Jaidi[1] and Mohamed Jamal Saadh[1]

*Address all correspondence to: prankishore1@gmail.com

1 Faculty of Pharmacy, Philadelphia University, Jordan

2 Pharmaceutical Chemistry Division, Shri Vishnu College of Pharmacy, Vishnupur, Andhra Pradesh, India

References

[1] Vane JR, Botting RM. Mechanism of action of anti-inflammatory drugs. Scandinavian Journal of Rheumatology. 1996;**102**:9-21. DOI: 10.3109/03009749609097226

[2] Vane JR, Botting RM. Anti-inflammatory drugs and their mechanism of action. Inflammation Research. 1998;**47**:S78-S87. DOI: 10.1007/s000110050284

[3] Smith RM, DeWitt DL, Garavito RM. CYCLOOXYGENASES: Structural, cellular, and molecular biology. Annual Review of Biochemistry. 2000;**69**:145-182. DOI: 10.1146/annurev.biochem.69.1.145

[4] Griswold DE. Adams JL. Constitutive cyclooxygenase (COX-1) and inducible cyclooxygenase (COX-2): Rationale for selective inhibition and progress to date. Medicinal Research Reviews. 1996;**16**:181-206. DOI: 10.1002/(SICI)1098-1128(199603)16:2<181::AID-MED3>3.0.CO;2-X

[5] Seibert K, Zhang Y, Leahy K, Hauser S, Masferrrer J, Perkins W, Lee L, Isakson P. Pharmacological and biochemical demonstration of the role of cyclooxygenase 2 in inflammation and pain. Proceedings National Academy of Sciences of the United State America. 1994;**91**:12013-12017

[6] Allison MC, Howatson AG, Torrance CJ, Lee FD, Russell RI. Gastrointestinal damage associated with the use of nonsteroidal anti-inflammatory drugs. The New England Journal of Medicine. 1992;**327**:749-754. DOI: 10.1056/NEJM199209103271101

[7] Clive DM, Stoff JS. Renal syndromes associated with nonsteroidal anti-inflammatory drugs. The New England Journal of Medicine. 1984;**310**:563-572. DOI: 10.1056/NEJM198403013100905

[8] FitzGerald GA. Coxibs and cardiovascular disease. The New England Journal of Medicine. 2004;**351**:1709-1711. DOI: 10.1056/NEJMp048288

[9] Kearney PM, Baigent C, Godwin J, Halls H, Emberson JR, Patrono C. Do selective cyclooxygenase-2 inhibitors and traditional nonsteroidal anti-inflammatory drugs increase the risk of atherothrombosis? Meta-analysis of randomised trials. BMJ. 2006;**332**:1302-1308. DOI: 10.1136/bmj.332.7553.1302

[10] Bresalier RS, Sandler RS, Quan H, Bolognese JA, Oxenius B, Horgan K, Lines C, Riddell R, Morton D, Lanas A, Konstam MA, Baron JA. Cardiovascular events associated with rofecoxib in a colorectal adenoma chemoprevention trial. The New England Journal of Medicine. 2005;**352**:1092-1102. DOI: 10.1056/NEJMoa050493

[11] Solomon SD, McMurray JJV, Pfeffer MA, Wittes J, Fowler R, Finn P, Anderson WF, Zauber A, Hawk E, Bertagnolli M. Cardiovascular risk associated with celecoxib in a clinical trial for colorectal adenoma prevention. The New England Journal of Medicine. 2005;**352**:1071-1080. DOI: 10.1056/NEJMoa050405

[12] Ritter JM, Harding I, Warren JB. Precaution, cyclooxygenase inhibition and cardiovascular risk. Trends in Pharmacological Sciences. 2009;**30**(10):503-508. DOI: 10.1016/j.tips.2009.07.007

[13] Zarraga IGE, Schwarz ER. Coxibs and heart disease. Journal of the American College of Cardiology. 2007;**49**:1-14. DOI: 10.1016/j.jacc.2006.10.003

[14] Hinz B, Renner B, Cheremina O, Besz D, Zolk O, Brune K. Lumiracoxib inhibits cyclooxygenase 2 completely at the 50 mg dose: Is liver toxicity avoidable by adequate dosing? Annals of the Rheumatic Diseases. 2009;**68**:289-291. DOI: 10.1136/ard.2008.092536

[15] Chakraborti AK, Sanjeev KG, Raj K, Hasim FM, Pradeep SJ. Progress in COX-2 Inhibitors: A journey so far. Current Medicinal Chemistry. 2010;**17**:1563-1593. DOI: 10.2174/092986710790979980

[16] Singh P, Mittal A. Current status of COX-2 inhibitors. Mini Reviews in Medicinal Chemistry. 2008;**8**:73-90. DOI: 10.2174/138955708783331577

[17] Gans KR, Galbraith W, Roman RJ, Haber SB, Kerr JS, Schmidt WK, Smith C, Hewes WE, Ackerman NR. Anti-inflammatory and safety profile of DuP 697, a novel orally effective prostaglandin synthesis inhibitor. Journal of Pharmacology and Experimental Therapeutics. 1990;**254**:180-187

[18] Prasit P, Wang Z, Briedeau C, Chan CC, Charleson S, Cromlish W, Ethier D, Evans JF, Ford-Hutchinson AW, Gauthier JY, Gordon R, Guay J, Gresser M, Kargman S, Kennedy B, Leblanc Y, Legar S, Mancini J, O'Neill GP, Ouellet M, Percival MD, Perrier H, Riendeau D, Rodger I, Tagari P, Therien M, Vikers P, Wong E, Xu LJ, Young RN, Zamboni R. The discovery of rofecoxib, [MK966, VIOXX,4-(4′-methylsulfonylphenyl)-3-phenyl-2(5H)-furanone], an orally active cyclooxygenase-2 inhibitor. Bioorganic & Medicinal Chemistry Letters. 1999;**9**:1773-1778. DOI: 10.1016/S0960-894X(99)00288-7

[19] Flower RJ. The development of COX-2 inhibitors. Nature Reviews Drug Discovery. 2003;**2**(3):179-191. DOI: 10.1038/nrd1034

[20] Marnett LJ, Kalgutkar AS. Cyclooxygenase 2 inhibitors: Discovery, selectivity and the future. Trends in Pharmacological Sciences. 1999;**20**(11):465-469. DOI: 10.1016/S0165-6147(99)01385-1

[21] Pran Kishore D, Rajwinder K, Balakumar C, Madhu B, Dilshad G, Venkat Rao K, Raghuram Rao A, Raghuprasad M. Synthesis, anti-inflammatory evaluation, and docking studies of some new thiazole derivatives. Medicinal Chemistry Research. 2014;**23**:2780-2792. DOI: 10.1007/s00044-013-0861-4

[22] Mamta SD, Pran Kishore D, Renu C, Tejvir S, Maninder K. Synthesis, evaluation and molecular docking studies of cycloalkyl/aryl-3,4,5-trimethylgallates as potent non-ulcerogenic and gastroprotective anti-inflammatory agents. Medicinal Chemistry Research. 2014;**23**:87-106. DOI: 10.1007/s00044-013-0620-6

[23] Pran Kishore D, Raghuprasad Maillabaram A, Raghuram RA, Mallikarjuna RP. Anti-inflammatory evaluation and docking studies of some new thienopyrimidines. Asian Journal of Chemistry. 2013;**25**(18):10583-10587. DOI: 10.14233/ajchem.2013.16184

[24] Alka B, Ruchika O, Pran Kishore D. Synthesis, evaluation and docking studies on 3-alkoxy-4-methanesulfonamido acetophenone derivatives as non-ulcerogenic anti-inflammatory agents. European Journal of Medicinal Chemistry. 2012;**49**:397-405. DOI: 10.1016/j.ejmech.2012.01.018

[25] Balakumar C, Lamba P, Pran Kishore D, Lakshminarayana B, Venkat Rao K, Rajwinder K, Raghuram Rao A, Shireesha B, Narsaiah B. Design, synthesis, biological evaluation and docking studies of some fluorinated fused-quinazolines as antiinflammatory agents. European Journal of Medicinal Chemistry. 2010;**45**:4904-4913. DOI: 10.1016/j.ejmech.2010.07.063

[26] Garavito RM, Malkowski MG, DeWitt DL. The structures of prostaglandin endoperoxide H synthases-1 and -2. Prostaglandins & Other Lipid Mediators. 2002;**68-69**:129-152. DOI: 10.1016/S0090-6980(02)00026-6

[27] Mbonye UR, Yuan C, Harris CE, Sidhu RS, Song I, Arakawa T, Smith WL. Two distinct pathways for cyclooxygenase-2 protein degradation. Journal of Biological Chemistry. 2008;**283**:8611-8623. DOI: 10.1074/jbc.M710137200

[28] Carol AR, Lawrence JM. Cyclooxygenases: Structural and functional insights. Journal of Lipid Research. 2009;**50**:S29-S34. DOI: 10.1194/jlr.R800042-JLR200

[29] Yuan C, Rieke CJ, Rimon G, Wingerd BA, Smith WL. Partnering between monomers of cyclooxygenase-2 homodimers. Proceedings of National Academy of Sciences of United States of America. 2006;**103**(16):6142-6147. DOI: 10.1073/pnas.0601805103

[30] Yuan C, Sidhu RS, Kuklev DV, Kado Y, Wada M, Song I, Smith WL. Cyclooxygenase Allosterism, fatty acid-mediated cross-talk between monomers of cyclooxygenase homodimers. The Journal of Biological Chemistry. 2009;**284**:10046-10055. DOI: 10.1074/jbc.M808634200

[31] Mitchener MM, Hermanson DJ, Shockley EM, Brown HA, Lindsley CW, Reese J, Rouzer CA, Lopez CF, Marnett LJ. Competition and allostery govern substrate selectivity of

cyclooxygenase-2. Proceedings of National Academy of Sciences of United States of America. 2015;**112**(40):12366–12371. DOI: 10.1073/pnas.1507307112

[32] Picot D, Loll PJ, Garavito RM. The X-ray crystal structure of the membrane protein prostaglandin H2 synthase-1. Nature. 1994;**367**:243-249.

[33] Kurumbail RG, Stevens AM, Gierse JK, McDonald JJ, Stegeman RA, Pak JY, Dildehaus D, Miyashiro JM, Penning TD, Seibert K, Isakson PC, Stallings WC. Structural basis for selective inhibition of cyclooxygenase-2 by anti-inflammatory agents. Nature. 1996;**384**:644-648.

[34] Lanzo CA, Sutin J, Rowlinson S, Talley J, Marnett LJ. Fluorescence quenching analysis of the association and dissociation of a diarylheterocycle to cyclooxygenase-1 and cyclooxygenase-2: Dynamic basis of cyclooxygenase-2 selectivity. Biochemistry. 2000;**39**(20):6228-6234. DOI: 10.1021/bi992761o

[35] Walker MC, Ravi GK, Kiefer JR, Morland KT, Koboldt CM, Isakson PC, Sebert K, Gierse JK. A three-step kinetic mechanism for selective inhibition of cyclo-oxygenase-2 by diarylheterocyclic inhibitors. Biochemical Journal. 2001;**357**(3):709-718. DOI: 10.1042/bj3570709

[36] Maestro, version 10.4. New York, NY: Schrödinger, LLC; 2015.

[37] Robert S, Carmen A, Susana GK, Javier LF, Modesto O. Theoretical studies on the inhibition mechanism of cyclooxygenase-2. Is there a unique recognition site? Journal of Medicinal Chemistry. 2003;**46**(8):1372-1382. DOI: 10.1021/jm0209376

[38] Vittorio L, Massimiliano B, Luciana M, Francesco LG, Andrea C, Ettore N, Michele P. Molecular basis of cyclooxygenase enzymes (COXs) selective inhibition. Proceedings of National Academy of Sciences of United States of America. 2010;**107**(12):5411-5416. DOI: 10.1073/pnas.0913377107

[39] Gilad R, Ranjinder SS, Adam LD, Jullia YL, Narayan PS, Chong Y, Ryan AF, Raymond CT, Benedict RL, William LS. Coxibs interfere with the action of aspirin by binding tightly to one monomer of cyclooxygenase-1. Proceedings of National Academy of Sciences of United States of America. 2010;**107**(1):28-33. DOI: 10.1073/pnas.0909765106

[40] So OY, Scarafia LE, Mak AY, Callan OH, Swinney DC. The dynamics of prostaglandin H synthases—Studies with prostaglandin H synthase-2 Y355F unmask mechanisms of time-dependent inhibition and allosteric activation. The Journal of Biological Chemistry. 1998;**273**:5801-5807. DOI: 10.1074/jbc.273.10.5801

[41] Selinsky BS, Gupta K, Sharkey CT, Loll PJ. Structural analysis of NSAID binding by prostaglandin H-2 synthase: Time-dependent and time-independent inhibitors elicit identical enzyme conformations. Biochemistry. 2001;**40**(17):5172-5180. DOI: 10.1021/bi010045s

[42] Orlando BJ, Malkowski MG. Crystal structure of rofecoxib bound to human cyclooxygenase-2. Acta Crystallographica Section F. 2016;**F72**:772-776. DOI: 10.1107/S2053230X16014230

[43] Marnett LJ. The COXIB experience: A look in the rearview mirror. Annual Review of Pharmacology Toxicology 2009;**49**:265-290. DOI: 10.1146/annurev.pharmtox.011008.145638

[44] Wang JL, Carter J, Kiefer JR, Kurumbail RG, Pawlitz JL, Brown D, Hartmann SJ, Graneto MJ, Seibert K, Talley JJ. The novel benzopyran class of selective cyclooxygenase-2 inhibitors-part I: The first clinical candidate. Bioorganic & Medicinal Chemistry Letters. 2010;**20**(23):7155-7158. DOI: 10.1016/J.BMCL.2010.07.053

[45] Lecomte M, Laneuville OJC, DeWitt DL, Smith WL. Acetylation of human prostaglandin endoperoxide synthase-2 (cyclooxygenase-2) by aspirin. The Journal of Biological Chemistry. 1994;**269**(18):13207-13215.

[46] Duggan KC, Walters MJ, Musee J, Harp JM, Kiefer JR, Oates JA, Marnett LJ. Molecular basis for cyclooxygenase inhibition by the nonsteroidal anti-inflammatory drug naproxen. Journal of Biological Chemistry. 2010;**285**:34950-34959. DOI: 10.1074/jbc.M110.162982

[47] Oriol L, Juan JP, Albert P, David M. Differential binding mode of diverse cyclooxygenase inhibitors. Journal of Molecular Graphics and Modelling. 2002;**20**(5):359-371. DOI: 10.1016/S1093-3263(01)00135-8

[48] Desiraju GR, Gopalakrishnan B, Jetti RKR, Nagaraju A, Raveendra D, Sarma JARP, Sobhia ME, Thilagavathi R. Computer-aided design of selective cox-2 inhibitors: Comparative molecular field analysis, comparative molecular similarity indices analysis, and docking studies of some 1,2-diarylimidazole derivatives. Journal of Medicinal Chemistry. 2002;**45**(22):4847-4857. DOI: 10.1021/jm020198t

[49] Adinarayana KPS, Reddy PA, Babu PA. Structural studies on docking selective COX-2 inhibitors. Journal of Bioinformatics & Research. 2012;**1**(1):21-26

[50] Jaspreet KD, Anith KS, Khushboo B., Shashank PK, Sukriti G, Abhinav G, Sundar D. Computational structure-based de novo design of hypothetical inhibitors against the anti-inflammatory target COX-2. Plos One. 2015;**10**(8):1-18. DOI: 10.1371/JOURNAL.PONE.0134691

[51] Wang JL, David L, Matthew JG, John S, Joseph RBH, Subo L, Jennifer LP, Ravi GK, Timothy M, John JT, James RK, Jeffery C. The novel benzopyran class of selective cyclooxygenase-2 inhibitors. Part 2: The second clinical candidate having a shorter and favorable human half-life. Bioorganic & Medicinal Chemistry Letters. 2010;**20**(23):7159-7163. DOI: 10.1016/J.BMCL.2010.07.054

Chapter 7

In Vivo Potential Anti-Inflammatory Activity of Extracts from *Calendula arvensis* (*CA*) Flowers

Abdulmalik Abdullah Abudunia, Rabie Kamal,
Nabeel Muhsen Ziad, Methaq Algabr,
Khadija Khedid, Katim Alaoui,
M'Hammed Ansar and Azeddine Ibrahimi

Additional information is available at the end of the chapter

http://dx.doi.org/10.5772/intechopen.68914

Abstract

Calendula arvensis (*CA*) had been reported in traditional Moroccan medicine to exhibit its extensive use to treat pain and inflammation. Therefore, the objective of this study was to evaluate the anti-inflammatory activity of *CA* flowers. The methanol, aqueous, and hexane extracts (ME, AE, and HE) were investigated for inflammatory effects by using two methods, namely, carrageenan and experimental trauma-induced hind paw edema in rats and using indomethacin (20 mg/kg body weight) as a standard drug. The results demonstrated that *Calendula Arvensis CA* extracts had significant anti-inflammatory activity where the HE at the doses of 300 and 500 mg/kg p.o. ($p < 0.001$) had the best significant reduction and inhibition of edema with 51.08, 71.33 and 63.38, 67.33% induced by carrageenan and on experimental trauma induced rat paw edema at third hour, respectively, and similar as compared with standard drug indomethacin 20 mg/kg body weight p.o. ($p < 0.001$). These results indicate that it could be suggested as contributory effects to the use of *CA* flowers in the management of inflammation and pain conditions.

Keywords: *Calendula arvensis*, anti-inflammatory activity, indomethacin, wistar male rats

1. Introduction

Morocco is known as the "emporium of medicinal plants" due to availability of several thousands of medicinal plants in the different bioclimatic zones, and it has favored the proliferation of more than 42,000 species of plants, divided into 150 families and 940 genuses [1–4].

Calendula arvensis (*CA*) (family asteraceae) [5] is found within a wide geographic distribution: central and southern Europe, northern Africa, southwestern Asia, and the Macaronesian region (the Azores Islands, the Madeira Islands, the Salvage Islands, the Canary Islands, and the Cape Verde Islands).

C. arvensis (*CA*) is an annual herb with tall reach to 10–50 cm, width of the leaves (5–20 mm), and is lance-shaped and borne on petioles from the slender. The inflorescence is a single flower head up to 4 cm wide, the color of the flowers are bright yellow to yellow-orange ray florets, and the fruit is an achene, which can take any of three shapes, including ring-shaped, that facilitate different methods of dispersal [6, 7].

Inflammation was described 2000 years ago by the four Latin words: rubor, calor, tumor, and dolor [8]. It is a healthy process resulting from some disturbances or disease and it is usually associated with pain as a secondary process resulting from the release of analgesic mediators: nonsteroidal anti-inflammatory drugs (NSAIDs), steroidal drugs, and immunosuppressant drugs, which have been used usually in the relief of inflammatory diseases by people around the world for a long time [9].

Most anti-inflammatory drugs and antiarthritic drugs have wide applications in clinical conditions [10], and they are associated with several side effects such as gastrointestinal tract complications, ulcers, and cardiovascular problems [11, 12]. Therefore, alternative therapies from natural resources are ventured throughout the world.

In the recent years, inflammation is one of the major target research areas among biomedical researchers, which includes various cellular processes (e.g., phagocytosis, chemotaxis, mitosis, and cell differentiation).

Thus, the aim of this study is to evaluate the anti-inflammatory effect of the extracts of the flowers of *CA* and, therefore, to determine the scientific basis for its use in traditional medicine in the treatment of inflammation.

2. Materials and methods

2.1. Sample collection and authentication

Flowers of *CA* were collected based on ethnopharmacological information from the villages around the region Rabat-Khemisset, with the agreement from the authorities and respecting the United Nations Convention of Biodiversity and with assistance of traditional medical practitioner. The plant was authenticated by Pr. M. Al-Saghir [botanist from Institute Scientific (IS) in Rabat], and a voucher specimen (N°RAB 78161) was deposited in the herbarium of the botany department.

2.2. Sample preparation and extraction

The aqueous extract (AE), 200 g of *CA* flowers powder was extracted in 500 mL of boiling water for 30 min. Then, the infusion was filtered and then freeze-dried [13].

The hexanolic and methanolic extracts (HE and ME) were, respectively, obtained by the method of soxhlet extraction of 200 g of *CA* flowers for 6 h in about 500 mL of solvents.

The filtrated extracts were evaporated using a rotator evaporator. After that, the extracts were concentrated to dryness and the residue was kept at 4°C [14].

2.3. Drugs and chemicals

The following drugs and chemicals were used in the studies: carrageenan (Sigma, St. Louis, Missouri, USA), PGE2 (Fluka Chemie AG), p-benzoquinone (Merck), indomethacin 20 mg/kg; all the plant extracts were dissolved in a mixture of arabic gum 5%, and then they were given to the test animals by oral mouth, and also the control group received the same treatment.

Indomethacin 20 mg/kg in 5% of gum arabic was used as the reference drug.

2.4. Animals

The study was performed on adult male rats (180–220 g), bred at the Laboratory of Pharmacology, Faculty of Medicine and Pharmacy of Rabat. All animals were kept in a room maintained under environmentally controlled conditions of 23 ′ 1°C and 12 h light–12 h dark cycle. The food was withdrawn on the day before the experiment; however, they were allowed free access to water and standard diet throughout the experiments, the animals were handled according to the prescribed ethical guidelines for laboratory animals.

2.5. Anti-inflammatory tests

In both methods, all animals were fasted 18 h before testing and received 5 mL of distilled water by gavages to minimize individual variations in response to the swelling of the paws. The left hind paw (LP) is not treated, and it is taken as control.

2.5.1. Carrageenan model

The carrageenan-induced hind paw edema model was used for the determination of anti-inflammatory activity [13–15]. Six animals were used for each extract dose, as well as the control and reference groups.

Note that 300 and 500 mg/kg doses were administered of extracts into the subplantar tissue of right hind paw of each rat that was injected with 35 μL of 30 mg/mL of freshly prepared carrageenan in physiological saline (0.9% NaCl). Note that 30 μL of saline was injected into subplantar tissue of left hind paw of control groups. Then, after the injection, the paw edema was measured at 1.5, 3, and 6 h.

Mean differences of treated groups were compared with the mean differences of the control group. The percentages of inhibition of inflammation were calculated according to the following formula:

$$\textbf{\% of inhibition} = \frac{\text{mean}\,[V_{left} - V_{right}]_{control} - [V_{left} - V_{right}]_{treated}}{[V_{left} - V_{right}]_{control}} * 100 \tag{1}$$

where V_{left} is the mean volume of edema on the left hind paw and V_{right} is the mean volume of edema on the right hind paw.

2.5.2. Experimental trauma model

This assay was determined as described by Riesterer and Jacques test [16].

The test groups of rats were given orally 300 and 500 mg/kg of each extract dose, the control group received 5 mL/kg of distilled water, and the standard group received the reference drug indomethacin 20 mg/kg.

One hour after oral administration of different substances dropping weight of 50 g onto the dorsum of the left hind paw of all animals. The right hind paw is not treated; it is taken as a witness. The difference volume of two paws was measured and taken as the edema value by using digital plethysmometer LE750 at 1 h 30 min, 3, and 6 h after induction of inflammation [17].

The percentages of inhibition of inflammation were calculated according to the following formula 2 where the mean differences of treated groups were compared with the mean differences of the control groups.

$$\textbf{\% of inhibition} = \frac{\text{mean}\,[V_{left} - V_{right}]_{control} - [V_{left} - V_{right}]_{treated}}{[V_{left} - V_{right}]_{control}} * 100 \tag{2}$$

where V_{left} is the mean volume of edema on the left hind paw and V_{right} is the mean volume of edema on the right hind paw.

2.5.3. Statistical analysis

The results are expressed as mean ' SEM and analyzed by one-way analysis of variance (ANOVA) followed by student's t-test. A value of $p < 0.001$ was considered significant.

3. Results and discussion

3.1. Carrageenan-induced rat paw edema

The results of the effect of the flowers *CA* extracts on carrageenan induced edema are shown in **Table 1** and **Figure 1** at doses of 300 and 500 mg/kg comparable to that of the control and standard drug indomethacin 20 mg/kg, p.o., and *CA* extracts exhibited significant ($p < 0.001$) anti-inflammatory activity as compared to the standard drug indomethacin 20 mg/kg (**Table 1** and **Figure 1**).

Treatment groups	Dose mg/kg p.o.	1 h 30 min	3 h 00min	6 h 00min
Control		0.458 ± 0.003	0.71 ± 0.009	0.55 ± 0.002
IND	20	0.06 ± 0.001*	0.113 ± 0.007*	0.135 ± 0.001*
EM	300	0.375 ± 0.001*	0.473 ± 0.002*	0.426 ± 0.005*
EM	500	0.318 ± 0.005*	0.363 ± 0.003*	0.325 ± 0.004*
EA	300	0.273 ± 0.003*	0.34 ± 0.005*	0.291 ± 0.001*
EA	500	0.2 ± 0.007*	0.251 ± 0.001*	0.235 ± 0.003*
EH	300	0.22 ± 0.005*	0.26 ± 0.007*	0.24 ± 0.001*
EH	500	0.123 ± 0.003*	0.158 ± 0.001*	0.136 ± 0.002*

Notes: Values are expressed as mean ± S.E.M. ($n = 6$), extracts of *CA* flowers, $^*p < 0.001$ statistically significant compared to the control and reference drug (indomethacin 20 mg/mL).

Table 1. Effect of extracts of *CA* flowers on carrageenan-induced rat paw edema.

The hexanolic extract showed maximum reduction and inhibition of edema by 51.08 and 71.43% at 300 and 500 mg/kg, respectively, compared to the aqeuose and methanolic extracts 48.26, 65.14, and 35.96, 52.63% respectively, and similar to standard drug indomethacin (20 mg/kg) by 72.36% during the same time (**Figure 1**).

3.2. Experimental trauma-induced rat paw edema

The effect of two doses 300 and 500 mg/kg p.o.of the *CA* extracts on experimental trauma-induced inflammation is shown in **Table 2** and **Figure 2**, and the results are comparable to

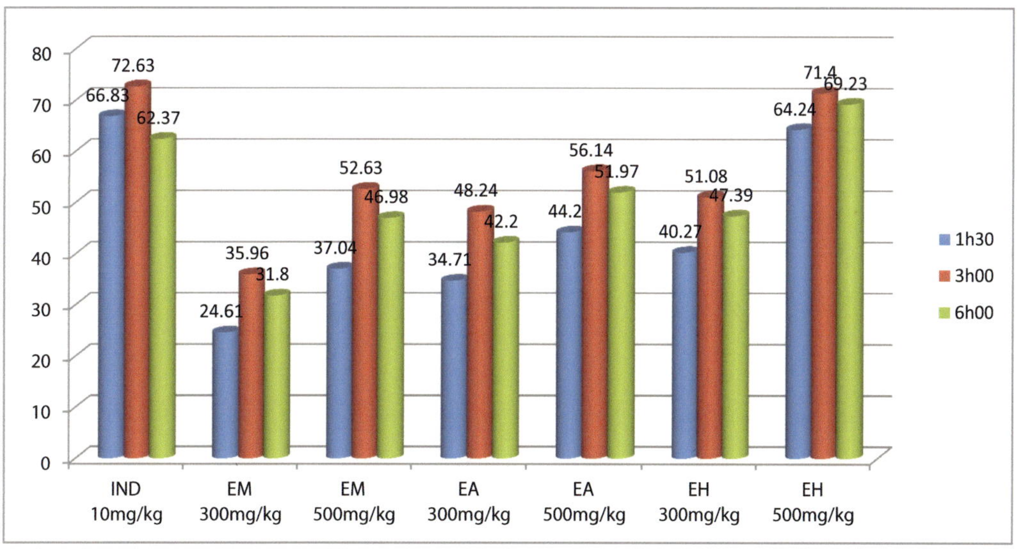

Figure 1. Percentage of inhibition of inflammation of extracts of *CA* flowers using carrageenan-induced rat paw edema.

Treatment groups	Dose mg/kg p.o.	1 h 30 min	3 h 00 min	6 h 00 min
Control		0.458 ± 0.003	0.71 ± 0.009	0.55 ± 0.002
IND	20	0.06 ± 0.001*	0.113 ± 0.007*	0.135 ± 0.001*
EM	300	0.375 ± 0.001*	0.473 ± 0.002*	0.426 ± 0.005*
EM	500	0.318 ± 0.005*	0.363 ± 0.003*	0.325 ± 0.004*
EA	300	0.273 ± 0.003*	0.34 ± 0.005*	0.291 ± 0.001*
EA	500	0.2 ± 0.007*	0.251 ± 0.001*	0.235 ± 0.003*
EH	300	0.22 ± 0.005*	0.26 ± 0.007*	0.24 ± 0.001*
EH	500	0.123 ± 0.003*	0.158 ± 0.001*	0.136 ± 0.002*

Notes: Values are expressed as mean ± S.E.M. ($n = 6$), extracts of *CA* flower, *$p < 0.001$ statistically significant compared to the control and reference drug (indomethacin 20 mg/mL).

Table 2. Effect of extracts of *CA* flowers on experimental trauma-induced rat paw edema.

that of the control and standard drug indomethacin 20 mg/kg, p.o. *CA* extracts exhibited significant ($p < 0.001$) anti-inflammatory activity as compared to the standard drug indomethacin 20 mg/kg (**Table 2** and **Figure 2**).

The hexanolic extract showed maximum reduction and inhibition of edema by 63.38 and 76.33% at 300 and 500 mg/kg, respectively, compared to the aqeuose and methanolic extracts

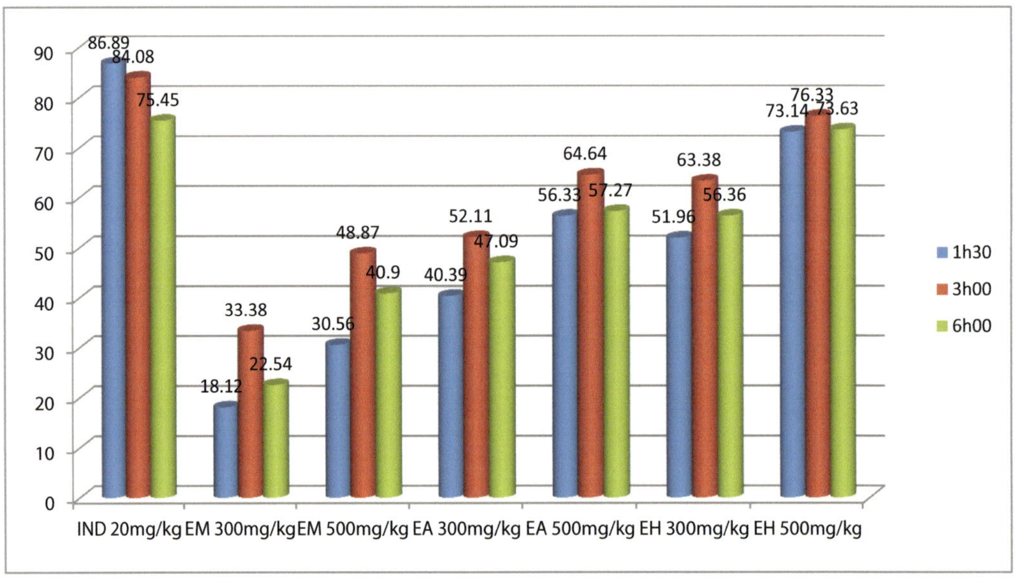

Figure 2. Percentage of inhibition of inflammation of extracts of *CA* flowers using experimental trauma-induced rat paw edema.

http://dx.doi.org/10.5772/intechopen.68914

52.11, 64.64 and 33.38, and 48.87%, respectively, and similar to standard drug indomethacin 20 mg/kg by 86.89% during the same time (**Figure 1**).

4. Discussion

Medicinal plant extracts have been used for thousands of years in the world by numerous civilizations.

Carrageenan-induced rat paw edema in rats is known to be sensitive to cyclo-oxygenase inhibitors and has been used to evaluate the effect of nonsteroidal anti-inflammatory agents, which primarily inhibit the cyclo-oxygenase involved in prostaglandin synthesis [18]. It plays a major role in the development of second phase of inflammatory reaction, which is measured at the third hour [19].

The anti-inflammatory activity of extracts of *CA* flowers is attributed to the present phytochemical constituents of these extracts, which include phenolic terpenoids, tannins, flavonoids; this results confirm our previously published results [20] and this is in agreement with many literature studies reporting that many plants containing these chemical classes of compounds have been reported to possess potent anti-inflammatory properties that act through inhibiting prostaglandin pathways [21].

5. Conclusion

Our study demonstrates significant anti-inflammatory activity where the hexanolic extract showed maximum inhibition of edema similar to the standard drug indomethacin (20 mg/kg) on carrageenan-induced paw edema and experimental trauma-induced rat paw edema in a dose-dependent fashion. Aqueous and methanolic extracts of *CA* flowers showed modest anti-inflammatory activity. This investigation suggests that *CA* flowers are a potential candidate for the discovery of new anti-inflammatory agents.

Acknowledgements

The authors would like to thank Pr. M. Al-Saghir [botanist from Institute Scientific (IS) in Rabat], for the botanical identification and collection of the plants used in this study. This work was carried out under intramural funding from the University of Mohammed the Vth of Rabat.

Conflicts of interest

The authors declare that they have no conflicts of interest.

Author details

Abdulmalik Abdullah Abudunia[1]*, Rabie Kamal[2], Nabeel Muhsen Ziad[3], Methaq Algabr[6], Khadija Khedid[5], Katim Alaoui[2], M'Hammed Ansar[4] and Azeddine Ibrahimi[1]

*Address all correspondence to: abdelmalek.dunia@um5s.net.ma

1 Department of Biotechnology Laboratory (Med-Biotech), Faculty of Medicine and Pharmacy, Mohammed V University, Rabat, Morocco

2 Department of Pharmacodynamic Research Team ERP, Laboratory of Pharmacology and Toxicology, Faculty of Medicine and Pharmacy, Mohamed V University, Rabat, Morocco

3 Department of Laboratory of Medicinal Chemistry, Faculty of Pharmacy, Sana'a University, Sana'a, Yemen

4 Department of Medicinal Chemistry Laboratory, Faculty of Medicine and Pharmacy, Mohammed V University, Rabat, Morocco

5 Department of Bacteriology, Institute National of Health (INH), Rabat, Morocco

6 Department of Laboratory of Chemistry, Faculty of Applied Sciences, University of Hajjah, Hajjah, Yemen

References

[1] Alnamer R, Alaoui K, Bouidida HE, Benjouad A, Cherrah Y. Toxicity and psychotropic activity of essential oils of *Rosmarinus officinalis* and *Lavandula officinalis* from Morocco. Journal of Biologically Active Products from Nature. 2012;**14**:262-272

[2] Alnamer R, Alaoui K, Bouidida HE, Benjouad A, Cherrah Y. Psychostimulant activity of *Rosmarinus officinalis* essential oils. Journal of Natural Products. 2012;**5**:83-92

[3] Alnamer R, Alaoui K, Bouidida HE, Benjouad A, Cherrah Y. Psychostimulants activity of *Rosmarinus officinalis L.* methanolic and aqueous extracts. Journal of Medicinal Plants Research. 2012;**6**(10):1860-1865

[4] Alnamer R, Alaoui K, Bouidida EH, Benjouad A, Cherrah Y. Sedative and hypnotic activities of the methanolic and aqueous extracts of *Lavandula officinalis* from Morocco. Advances in Pharmacological Sciences. 2012;**2012**:5

[5] Heyn CC, Joel A. Reproductive relationships between annual species of *Calendula* (Compositae). Plant Systematics and Evolution. 1983;**143**:311-329

[6] Ruiz de Clavijo E. The reproductive strategies of the heterocarpic annual *Calendula arvensis* (Asteraceae). Acta Oecologica. 2005;**28**:2119-2126

[7] Messina, Nino (2010). "Calendula arvensis". Actaplantarum. Retrieved 21 January 2015

[8] Chatterjee A, Sen B, Das S, Chatterjee TK. Antiinflammatory and analgesic activity of methanolic extract of medicinal plant *Rhodiola roseal* rhizomes. International Journal of Pharma Research & Review. 2015;**4**(2):1-8

[9] Alwashli A, Al-sobarry M, Alnamer R, Cherrah Y, Alaoui K. Analgesic and anti inflammatory activities of *Boswellia elongata balf* methanolic extracts, as endemic plants in Yemen. Journal of Biologically Active Products from Nature. 2012;**2**(2):90-98

[10] Gaffo A, Saag KG, Curtis JR. Treatment of rheumatoid arthritis. American Journal of Health-System Pharmacy. 2006;**63**:2451-2465

[11] Singh G, Ramey DR, Morfeld D, Shi H, Hatoum HT, et al. Gastrointestinal tract complications of nonsteroidal antiinflammatory drug treatment in rheumatoid arthritis: A prospective observational cohort study. Archives of Internal Medicine. 1996;**156**:1530-1536

[12] Emmanuel, J.H. & Montgomery, R.D. Gastric ulcer and anti-arthritic drugs. Postgraduate Medical Journal, 1971;**47**:227-232.

[13] J.B. Harborne: Phytochemical Methods. A guide to modern techniques of plant analysis. 2nd. Ed. Chapman and Hall ltd., London, New York 1984;288

[14] Rudzik AD, Hester JB, Tang AH, Staw RN, Friis W, editors. The Benzodiazepines. New York, USA: Raven Press; 1973

[15] Yamada K, Mimaki Y, Sashida Y. Effects of inhaling the vapor of Lavandula burnatii super-derived essential oil and linalool on plasma adrenocorticotropic hormone (ACTH), catecholamine and gonadotropin levels in experimental menopausal female rats. Biological and Pharmaceutical Bulletin. 2005;**28**(2):378-379

[16] Bignotto L, Rocha J, Sepodes B, et al. Antiinflammatory effect of lycopene on carrageenan-induced paw edema and hepatic ischaemia-reperfusion in the rat. British Journal of Nutrition. 2009;**102**(1):126-133

[17] Sonavane GS, Sarveiya VP, Kasture VS, Kasture SB. Anxiogenic activity of *Myristica fragrans* seeds. Pharmacology Biochemistry and Behavior. 2002;**71**(1-2):239-244

[18] Crunkhorn P, Meacock SC. Mediators of the inflammation induced in the rat paw by carrageenan. British Journal of Pharmacology. 1971;**42**:392-402

[19] Di Rosa M, Willoughby DA. Screens for antiinflammatory drugs. Journal of Pharmacy and Pharmacology. 1971;**23**:2978

[20] Abudunia AM, et al. Anticandidal, antibacterial, cytotoxic and antioxidant activities of *Calendula arvensis* flowers. Journal De Mycologie Médicale. 2016

[21] Oyekunle AO, Idowu AO. Antiinflammatory activity of methanolic extract of *Cnidoscolous aconitifolius* leaves in laboratory rodents. Journal of Chemical, Biological and Physical Sciences. 2012;**2**(2):770-774

Chapter 8

Apoptotic Effects of Etodolac in Breast Cancer Cell Cultures

Oya Orun, Pınar Mega Tiber and
Sevgi Koçyiğit Sevinç

Additional information is available at the end of the chapter

http://dx.doi.org/10.5772/67855

Abstract

Nonsteroidal anti-inflammatory drugs (NSAIDs) are commonly used as anti-inflammatory and analgesic agents. This family of drugs suppresses prostaglandin synthesis through inhibition of cyclooxygenase (COX) enzymes. Recent studies displayed that anti-carcinogenic actions of these drugs are mediated by COX-2 enzyme. Currently, there is intense research on COX-2 inhibitors as therapeutic targets. Etodolac is not perfectly selective but shows 'preferential selectivity' for COX-2. Here, in this study, we wanted to take gene expression snapshots of several apoptotic proteins under different conditions of drug exposure. The aim, therefore, focused to determine differential effects of etodolac on the regulation of apoptotic genes in hormone-responsive MCF-7 and triple-negative MDA-MB-231 cancer cell lines. Our data suggest that MDA-MB-231 is more responsive to etodolac exposure. Cell proliferation and apoptosis consistently regulated upon drug addiction. Furthermore, COX-2/HER2 was explicitly an up-regulated, phosphorylated form of Bad accumulated and anti-apoptotic proteins SAG and survivin increased in both transcriptional and translational levels. Changes in mitochondrial Bcl-2 family proteins were moderate and pro- and anti-apoptotic proteins showed similar levels of regulation in both cell lines. We believe that these findings would be supportive for future studies targeting etodolac-based therapies, as it reveals apoptotic factors differentially regulated in hormone-responsive and invasive cell lines.

Keywords: apoptosis, MCF-7, MDA-MB-231, MTT, Bad, SAG

1. Introduction

Nonsteroidal anti-inflammatory drugs (NSAIDs), regularly used for their anti-inflammatory and analgesic effects, were shown to have potency for cancer prevention as well [1, 2]. This family of drugs suppresses prostaglandin synthesis through inhibition of cyclooxygenase (COX) enzymes. COX enzymes have two isoforms COX-1 and COX-2, with a recent addition of a splice variant of COX-1, COX-3, which is not functional in humans. COX-1 is commonly expressed in body, showing constitutive activation. COX-2, on the other hand, is hardly detectable in normal conditions but is induced upon stimulation by mitogenic agents, cytokines, growth factors, and so on. Later reports, however, demonstrated that COX-2 is also constitutively expressed in basal levels at several tissues including gastric mucosa, developing brain or kidney [3–5].

COX isoforms catalyse prostaglandin G/H (PGG2/PGH2) synthesis from arachidonic acid, and these prostaglandins are then converted to stable forms like PGD2, PGE2, PGF2, prostacyclin (PGI2) or thromboxane A2 (TXA2) depending on the cell type. Inhibition of COX enzymes, therefore, could result in improper prostaglandin activity, which in turn may cause different side effects. Since COX-1 was mostly expressed in gastrointestinal tract (GI), intestinal side effects of NSAIDs were suggested to decline if selective COX-2 inhibitors were used. A detailed discussion about the role of COX enzymes in GI damage can be found in a review by Lazzaroni et al. [6].

A wide range of COX-2 inhibitors (coxibs) were introduced to the market. Soon after clinical approval and usage, most of these drugs were withdrawn due to the emerging new side effects. Selective COX-2 inhibition partly reduced GI-related pathologies, but they were marked for their adverse effects in cardiovascular (CV) system. Regulation of blood coagulation involves the action of COX enzymes: COX-1 in platelets produces TXA2, and COX-2 in endothelial cells produces PGI2, achieving a balance between thrombotic/anti-thrombotic activities [7]. Drugs targeting one of the enzymes specifically could alter this balance and can cause bleeding or thrombosis. In this context, prevalent COX isoform in vascular endothelium was also a point of debate and a recent report showed that it is the COX-1, rather than COX-2, that is responsible for prostacyclin release in these cells [8]. Altogether, these findings imply necessity of further work on the side effects of COX-2 inhibitors.

Early reports about the role of NSAIDs in cancer were from the studies on colorectal cancer (CRC). Inducible form of COX enzymes, namely COX-2, was found to be elevated in colorectal cancer patients and early polyp formations were preceded by COX-2 induction [9]. Regular use of NSAIDs reportedly reduced CRC occurrence in 30–50%, mostly by COX inhibition, though later studies revealed that COX-2 inhibitors could also act on COX-independent pathways [2, 10]. These studies were further confirmed by many others and in different types of cancers like prostate, breast or lung cancers [11–13].

COX-2 is the main form participating in PGE2 production. When its activity is suppressed, protein expression is up-regulated [14]. Since there is strong evidence that COX-2 expression-related PGE2 increase acts on tumourigenesis and possible side effects could be reduced by targeting molecular downstream effectors taking part in this pathway such as cell cycle regulation, inhibiting proliferation and inducing apoptosis.

Presented study summarizes current knowledge available on various coxib agents in molecular level. Besides, it focuses on the molecular effects of etodolac in cancer cells. As a part of our study, we are testing various etodolac derivatives synthesized by our collaborators. Etodolac has different structural characteristic than other coxibs, in that it has no sulphonyl, sulphonamide or sulphone groups to facilitate COX-2 binding. Its toxicity and relative selectivity for COX-2 are low, and although there are numerous studies about its anti-cancerogenic activity, dose-response relationship on various cancer cell lines and molecular downstream effectors was not well documented. Here, we present our preliminary results on the expression changes of various apoptotic proteins between hormone responsive and nonresponsive breast cancer cell lines under different doses and points.

2. COX-2 inhibitors and their biological effects

2.1. COX-2 inhibitors (coxibs) in common use

Specific COX-2 inhibitors rofecoxib and valdecoxib were withdrawn from the market due to their cardiovascular side effects [15]. Celecoxib, brand name Celebrex, presented to the market by Pfizer, is still in use, with precaution for possible cardiovascular thrombotic events. In addition to its anti-inflammatory and analgesic properties, celecoxib is also known to reduce premalignant adenomatous polyps and affects signalling pathways involved in malignant transformation in tumours, but not in normal tissues [16]. Celecoxib showed COX-1/COX-2 ratio of 30 in IC50 values, meaning that it has 30 times more potency at inhibiting COX-2 with respect to COX-1. Rofecoxib, was introduced to the market at the same time, has nearly 272-fold potency in COX-2 selectivity. This higher selectivity on COX-2 inhibition resulted in more severe adverse effects of the drug, and its use was banned by Food and Drug Administration (FDA).

Etoricoxib is developed by Merck & Co. It is approved in many countries worldwide, with the exception of US. Selectivity of this drug for COX-2 is nearly 100-fold more than COX-1 [17]. Parecoxib is another COX-2 inhibitor drug introduced to the market. Since parecoxib is a prodrug of valdecoxib, it has similar pharmacodynamic properties as valdecoxib, which have a COX-1/COX-2 IC50 ratio of around 60, 2–2.5-fold higher than that of celecoxib, and it has no anti-thrombotic activity. Both drugs were not approved by the Food and Drug Administration (FDA) yet, but they are available in Europe and many other countries. Lumiracoxib (Novartis AG) is one of the most selective COX-2 inhibitors with significant reduction in gastrointestinal side effects [18]. Though it is being approved in more than 50 countries, it was not approved by FDA.

Several randomized clinical studies suggest that the novel coxibs have comparable efficacy to nonselective NSAIDs in the treatment of osteoarthritis, rheumatoid arthritis and acute pain, but they share similar renal side effects. The apparent dose dependence of renal toxicity may limit the use of higher doses of the novel coxibs for improved efficacy. Large-size randomized clinical trials are ongoing to define the gastrointestinal and cardiovascular safety of the novel coxibs.

Etodolac is one of the first NSAIDs approved by FDA. It has been grouped in family showing 'preferential selectivity' for COX-2 together with meloxicam and nimesulide [19]. It has approximately threefold higher selectivity for COX-2, but full dose could be inhibitory for COX-1, too.

2.2. COX-2/PGE2 signalling pathway

To prevent adverse side effects of NSAIDs and to better describe their anti-carcinogenic properties, it is important to clarify COX-2-related signalling pathways, especially on proliferation, cell cycle and apoptosis. Since most of their anti-carcinogenic effects are produced by COX-2/PGE2 regulation, direct intervention with the downstream players could be a promising approach to reduce unwanted side effects.

Downstream targets of PGE2 are four different G-protein-coupled receptors (EP1, EP2, EP3 and EP4) on the membrane, each initiating different signalling systems. The EP1 receptor is coupled to the Gαq protein subunit that activates phosphoinositide signalling through phospholipase C (PLC). PLC hydrolyses phosphatidylinositol 4,5-bisphosphate (PIP2) to generate the secondary messengers inositol 1,4,5-triphosphate (IP3) and diacylglycerol (DAG) This signalling pathway regulates intracellular calcium through PLC/IP3 and activates protein kinase C (PKC) through DAG. Clinical observations do not support any strict correlation between EP1 and cancer. However, since the activation of PLC ultimately leads to the activation of PKC, gene transcription would be effected due to mitogen-activated protein (MAP) kinase, nuclear factor-kappaB (NFκB) or Bcl2/Bad pro-apoptotic pathways [20–22]. EP1 was also shown to contribute to the development of UVB- or chemically induced skin cancers. UVB-induced squamous cell carcinomas display higher levels of EP1 expression than uninvolved skin [23]. Consistent with these conclusions is that the topical application of a selective EP1 antagonist protects against UVB-induced tumours [24].

While EP1 seems to have a secondary role in tumourigenesis, EP2-EP4 receptors obviously effect major cancer-signalling pathways. Secondary messenger systems like Gαs-cAMP-ERK signalling activated by EP2 or Ras/MAPK/ERK signalling activated by EP4 could affect cellular functions like differentiation, cell survival, cell growth or proliferation and apoptosis. EP2 also works through PI3K/Akt system together with axin and APC, leading to the accumulation of unphosphorylated form of β-catenin in the cytoplasm. The result would be a series of events initiated by transcription factors to yield cell proliferation, survival or angiogenesis [20].

A recent study reported interesting relation between PGE2 and insulin-like growth factor (IGF-1)/Akt/mTORC1-signalling pathway in recovering effects of obesity in pancreatic cancer cells. The study reveals that PGE2-stimulated mTORC1 activation occurs not through Akt but rather through cooperative action of EP4/cAMP/PKA and EP1/Ca2+ pathways [25].

EP2 positively and EP3 negatively regulate adenylate cyclase mediated by heterotrimeric G-proteins G-alphas or G-alphai, respectively. Resultant activation/deactivation of protein kinase A changes transcription factor activities of CREB and ERK1/2 through phosphorylation, which are correlated with phosphorylation of Bad or activation of cyclin D1, COX-2 and VEGF, respectively.

EP4 leads to the activation of adenylate cyclase, cAMP formation, activation of MAPK signalling, with an end point of CREB activation. This, in turn, causes the rise in Bcl-2 levels and inhibition of p53-induced apoptosis [26, 27].

2.3. Molecular pathway studies on coxibs

Etodolac-induced apoptosis was studied in Burkitt's lymphoma cells, and it was shown that the induction is higher with respect to meloxicam, a drug classified in the 'preferential selective' COX-2 inhibitors, such as etodolac [10]. In this study, the treatment of cell with 100 μM etodolac was sufficient to reduce Bcl-2, Bcl-xL, cIAP-1 and survivin, and cleaved Procaspase-9, -3 and PARP in a dose-dependent manner. Since these cells do not express COX-2 enzyme, observed effects might be following a COX-2-independent pathway. Down-regulation of Bcl-2 was also reported in prostate cancer cell lines. In accordance with Kobayashi's report, there was no change in COX-2 levels after etodolac treatment and growth inhibition was correlated with hormone sensitivity. On the other hand, induction of apoptosis by celecoxib did not show any hormone dependency and progressed through Akt regulation, instead of Bcl-2 [11, 28].

Bcl-2, an antiapoptotic protein, prevents induction of apoptosis by sequestering BH-3 only proteins like Bim, Bid, NOXA, PUMA, phosphorylated Bad or BNIP. These BH3-only proteins can either activate (directly or indirectly) Bax or Bak proteins, which are located at the mitochondrial outer membrane and change permeabilization or they inactivate anti-apoptotic Bcl-2 family members [29]. When there is an apoptotic stimulus, BH3-only proteins are up-regulated and they can directly act on Bax and Bak, initiating cytochrome c release through VDAC (voltage-dependent anion channel). In addition to direct activator BH-3-only proteins, sensitizer BH-3 group, such as Bad, NOXA or BNIP3, can release activators from anti-apoptotic BH1-4 proteins and initiate apoptosis through an indirect pathway [30, 31]. PUMA, an activator of BH3 protein, and NOXA, a sensitizer, both are found to be expressed in a p53-dependent manner.

Molecular studies to understand COX-2 inhibitors' action mostly concentrated on two specific coxibs, celecoxib and rofecoxib. In HT-29 cells, celecoxib was found to reduce p38 and p55 MAPK phosphorylation, together with a reduction in adhesion molecules ICAM-1 and VCAM-1 [32]. Data indicated that there is an induction of pro-apoptotic response (Bax and Bid) in a dose-time-dependent manner. Global transcription profiling in colon cancers implied modulations on the genes related to cell cycle and apoptosis, but these changes were mostly observed in both COX-2 (+) and (-) cell lines [33]. Celecoxib induces cell cycle arrest at G1-phase, together with decreases in the inhibition of various cyclin expressions. Celecoxib can inhibit protein kinase B (PKB/Akt) or its upstream kinase phosphoinositide-dependent kinase 1 (PDK-1) [34, 35]. Partial inhibition of PKB/Akt results in a relative activation of cell cycle inhibitors p21 and p27, which can cause the partial inactivation of cyclin-CDK complexes. However, a detailed mechanism has not been elucidated, since there was no change in the expressions of p21 and p27, cyclins or in the phosphorylation of CDK complexes [36].

Cell cycle gene profiling was conducted in normal breast epithelial cells, where 96 genes in p53 pathway were studied under two different doses of etodolac (0.5 and 2 mM) for 48 h [37]. Prominent regulation was observed in ATM, CCND2 (Cyclin D2), CCNF (Cyclin F), CDC20 (p55cdc), CDKIN1A (p21) and RAD50. Apoptotic protein BAX was found to be down-regulated only after 2-mM application.

3. Methods

3.1. Cell viability assay

Cell viability was determined using Cell Proliferation Kit I (MTT) (Roche) according to the manufacturer's instructions. Briefly, cells were seeded into 96-well plates (10^4 cells/well) and incubated at 37°C in CO_2 incubator for 24 h. The next day, appropriate doses of drug were added and cells were further incubated for 24 or 48 h. MTT of 10 μL was added to each well for an additional 4 h. The precipitated formazan was dissolved in 100 μL of 10% SDS, and the absorbance was taken at 570 nm [38].

3.2. Assays for apoptosis

Tali™ Image-Based Apoptosis Kit utilizing Annexin V/propidium iodide (PI) binding was used to assess apoptotic cells (green fluorescence), dead cells (red and yellow fluorescence) and live cells (no fluorescence). The Tali™ Image-Based Cytometer has two in-built fluorescence channels: (1) green channel to measure V-Alexa Fluor® 488, using 458-nm excitation and 525/20-nm emission filters and (2) red channel to measure propidium iodide, using 530-nm excitation and 585-nm longpass emission filters. The alterations in permeability of mitochondrial membrane were studied using JC-1 Mitochondrial Membrane Potential Kit (Abnova). All assays were performed according to the manufacturer's protocols. Spectral readout was done using Synergy H1 Multi-Mode Microplate Reader (BioTek).

3.3. Real-time PCR analysis

Total RNA was purified using the RNeasy Plus Mini Kit (Qiagen) containing g-eliminator columns. Purity and quantification of products were tested through absorbance measurements and gel imaging. RNAs of 1 μg were reverse transcribed to cDNAs using Transcriptor High Fidelity cDNA Synthesis Kit (Roche) according to the manufacturer's guidelines. Real-time PCR was applied using LightCycler 480 SYBR Green I Master Kit (Roche). Custom

http://dx.doi.org/10.5772/67855

plate involving primers for 16 genes of interest was designed and produced by Qiagen. Fold changes were evaluated through on-site web application of the same company.

3.4. Western blot

Cells were lysed with 1× RIPA buffer (50 mM Tris-HCl, pH 8.0, 150 mM NaCl, 1% NP40, 0.5% Na-deoxycholate, 0.1% SDS) containing protease inhibitor cocktail (Complete, EDTA-free Protease Inhibitor Cocktail Tablets, Roche) and 10 mM phosphatase inhibitor sodium fluoride (Santa Cruz, SC-24988B). Proteins of 40 μg were resolved by SDS-PAGE and transferred to PVDF membranes. Membranes were incubated with primary and secondary antibodies after optimization. RNF7/SAG (Novus Biologicals, NBP1-85594), survivin (Novus Biologicals, NB500-201H) and phosphorylated Bad (pSer112) (Novus Biologicals, NB100-81807) were polyclonal clones produced in rabbit. Beta-actin (Novus Biologicals, NB600-501) was monoclonal antibody produced in mouse. Detection was performed using chemiluminescent substrates for HRP (Western Bright ECL-Advansta, K-12045-050) and Celvin S Chemiluminescence Imaging System (BioStep).

4. Results

4.1. Effects of etodolac on the proliferation of breast cancer cell cultures

The role of COX-2 inhibitors in tumourigenesis was a focus of interest in recent years. The most commonly used, FDA-approved, COX-2 inhibitor in market is celecoxib. A recent study presented full effects of celecoxib both *in vivo* and *in vitro* on breast cancer cells [39]. Growth inhibitory effects of celecoxib were clearly observable between ranges 10 and 40 μM, especially after 72- and 96-h incubations.

Etodolac is another approved COX-2 inhibitor being used generally as adjuvant to chemotherapeutic applications. Early studies on etodolac were performed in colorectal cancers, and later it was tested in various other types such as liver, lung or prostate. In our study, cytotoxicity of etodolac was determined using MTT assay in two breast cancer cell lines, one of which is known for its good prognosis (MCF-7) and the other for its malignant, invasive properties (MDA-MB-231). Proliferative effects of etodolac were insignificant at low concentrations (0–100 μM) in both cell lines. When concentrations were raised to 0.5 or 1 mM, cell viability in both cell lines was considerably decreased (**Figure 1A**). Etodolac was less effective in MCF-7, but there was a regular dose-response relation in MDA-MB-231 cells at the end of 48 h (**Figure 1B**). A good correlation was observed with the study where regular HT-29 was compared with the invasive-type colon cancer cell line HT-29/Inv3 by Chen et al., where invasive type was found to be more susceptible to the effect of etodolac with a relative IC50 values of 0.5 versus 1.88 mM for other cell lines [40]. In our case, IC50 value for MDA-MB-231 was found to be 0.69 mM, while no approximation was available for MCF-7.

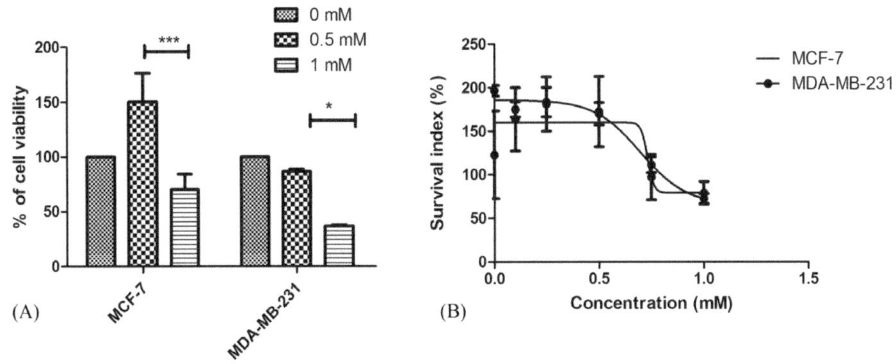

Figure 1. Cell viability effect of etodolac on breast cancer cell lines. (A) Decrease in cell viability upon 0.5 and 1 mM etodolac addition. Each bar represents the mean ± SD of three independent experiments. Two-way ANOVA was applied for each pair. *$P < 0.05$, ***$P < 0.001$. (B) Dose-response curve for MCF-7 and MDA-MB-231 cells treated with increasing concentration of etodolac (100, 250, 500, 750 and 1000 μM) for 48 h.

4.2. Determination of apoptosis

There was no detectable apoptotic effect of etodolac at low doses, in accordance with our observations from MTT assays. When concentrations were raised to mM range, apoptosis was detectable through changes in mitochondrial membrane potential (**Figure 2A**). Apoptotic effect of etodolac was more prominent in MDA-MB-231 cells at the end of 48 h.

Apoptosis was further confirmed with Annexin V/PI staining using Tali™ Apoptosis Kit (Thermo Fisher Scientific) (**Figure 2B**).

4.3. Transcriptional profiling of apoptotic proteins of interest

To understand molecular mechanisms underlying observed apoptotic effects of etodolac and to clarify COX-2 dependency of anti-carcinogenic responses, regulatory changes in apoptotic pathways were investigated at molecular level. To achieve this, 10^5–10^6 cells were collected for

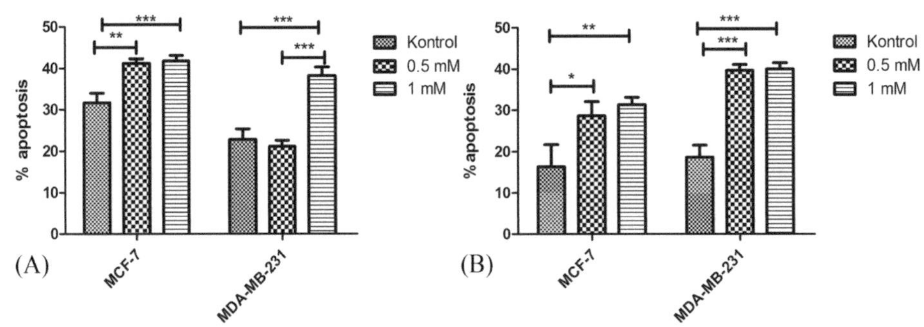

Figure 2. Effect of etodolac on apoptosis in MCF-7 and MDA-MB-231 cell lines. (A) The ratio of apoptotic to health cells at the end of 48-h incubation period was quantified by JC-1 staining with or without etodolac. (B) Apoptotic/dead cells were counted following Annexin V/PI staining using Tali™ Apoptosis Kit as described in Methods. Two-way ANOVA was applied for each pair. *$P < 0.05$; **$P < 0.01$; ***$P < 0.001$.

real-time and Western blot analyses as described in Section 3. Cell pellets were stored at −80°C to the day of experiments. Custom-designed 96-well-plate-containing primers for the genes of interest were purchased from Qiagen-SAB Bioscience. Fold changes were calculated from Ct values, using delta-delta Ct method. All values were normalized to GADPH expression and calculated with respect to non-drugged controls (**Table 1**).

Genes over-expressed in			**Genes under-expressed in**		
Sample name	**Gene symbol (mM)**	**Fold regulation***	**Sample name**	**Gene symbol (mM)**	**Fold regulation**
24 h					
MCF-7			**MCF-7**		
BAD1	0.5	++	**BCL2L11**	0.5	–
	1	++		1	–
BAK1	0.5	+	**PMAIP1**	0.5	–
	1	+			
BAX	0.5	++	**HIF1A**	0.5	–
	1	+			
BID	0.5	+	**TP53**	0.5	–
	1	+		1	–
MB231					
COX2	0.5	++			
	1	+			
ERBB2	0.5	++			
	1	++			
BAX	0.5	+			
	1	+			
BID	0.5	+			
	1	+			
HIF1A	0.5	+			
TP53	0.5	+			
	1	+			
48 h					
MCF-7			**MCF-7**		
ERBB2	0.5	+	**BAD1**	0.5	–
			BAK1	0.5	–
MB231			**BCL2L11**	0.5	–
COX2	0.5	++	**BAX**	1	–

Genes over-expressed in			Genes under-expressed in		
Sample name	**Gene symbol (mM)**	**Fold regulation***	**Sample name**	**Gene symbol (mM)**	**Fold regulation**
ERBB2	0.5	++	**SAG**	0.5	–
BCL2L11	0.5	++	**Survivin**	0.5	–
SAG	0.5	++	**TP53**	0.5	–

* + and – signs were used for up- and down-regulations, respectively. Fold regulations >10 were signified using two marks.

Table 1. Fold changes after 24- and 48-h incubation periods upon addition of 0.5 and 1 mM etodolac into cultures.

All analyses were made through Qiagen website facility provided for data analysis.

Etodolac induced an early increase in pro-apoptotic proteins Bad1, Bak1, Bax and Bid gene expression, accompanied by Bcl-2 down-regulation for both concentrations in MCF-7 cells. These changes were seen to decline as period was extended to 48 h. Another prompt response was the up-regulation of HER-2 and COX-2 in MDA-MB-231 cells. There was a remarkable up-regulation of anti-apoptotic SAG protein after 48-h incubation in MDA-MB-231 cells, parallel to BCL2L11 (**Figure 3A** and **B**).

4.4. Etodolac promoted anti-apoptotic pathways in MDA-MB-231 cells

In translational level, phosphorylated form of Bad has slightly increased upon etodolac addition in MDA-MB-231 cells. SAG and survivin have also increased similarly in this cell line, in a dose- and time-dependent manner (**Figure 4A–C**).

Low drug concentrations were also examined in long-term culturing to see differences in relation to various dose-time applications. Etodolac was added into cultures at 100 and 200 μM concentrations. Neither cell proliferation nor cell deaths were significantly affected under these concentrations (data not shown). Real-time PCR analysis implicated that protein expressions were only moderately regulated in transcriptional level for all, except a consistent increase in anti-apoptotic proteins, including SAG, in invasive MDA-MB-231 cells (**Figure 5A** and **B**).

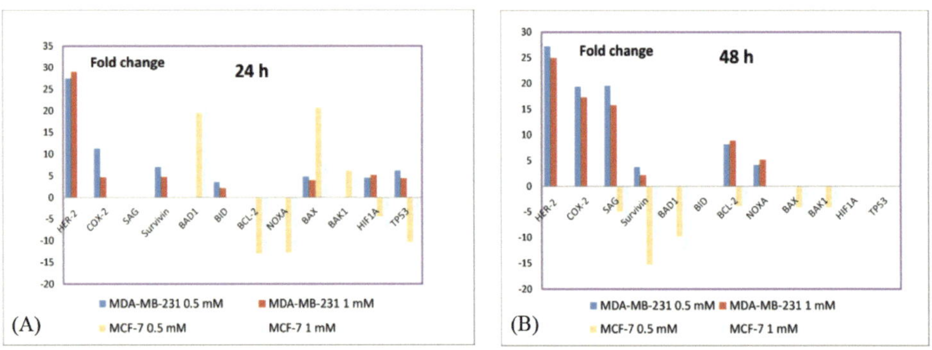

Figure 3. Differential expression of 12 genes chosen in relation to COX-2/apoptotic pathway. Fold changes were relative to control cells treated with DMSO after (A) 24 h and (B) 48 h. All expressions were normalized to GAPDH expression of corresponding cell line.

http://dx.doi.org/10.5772/67855

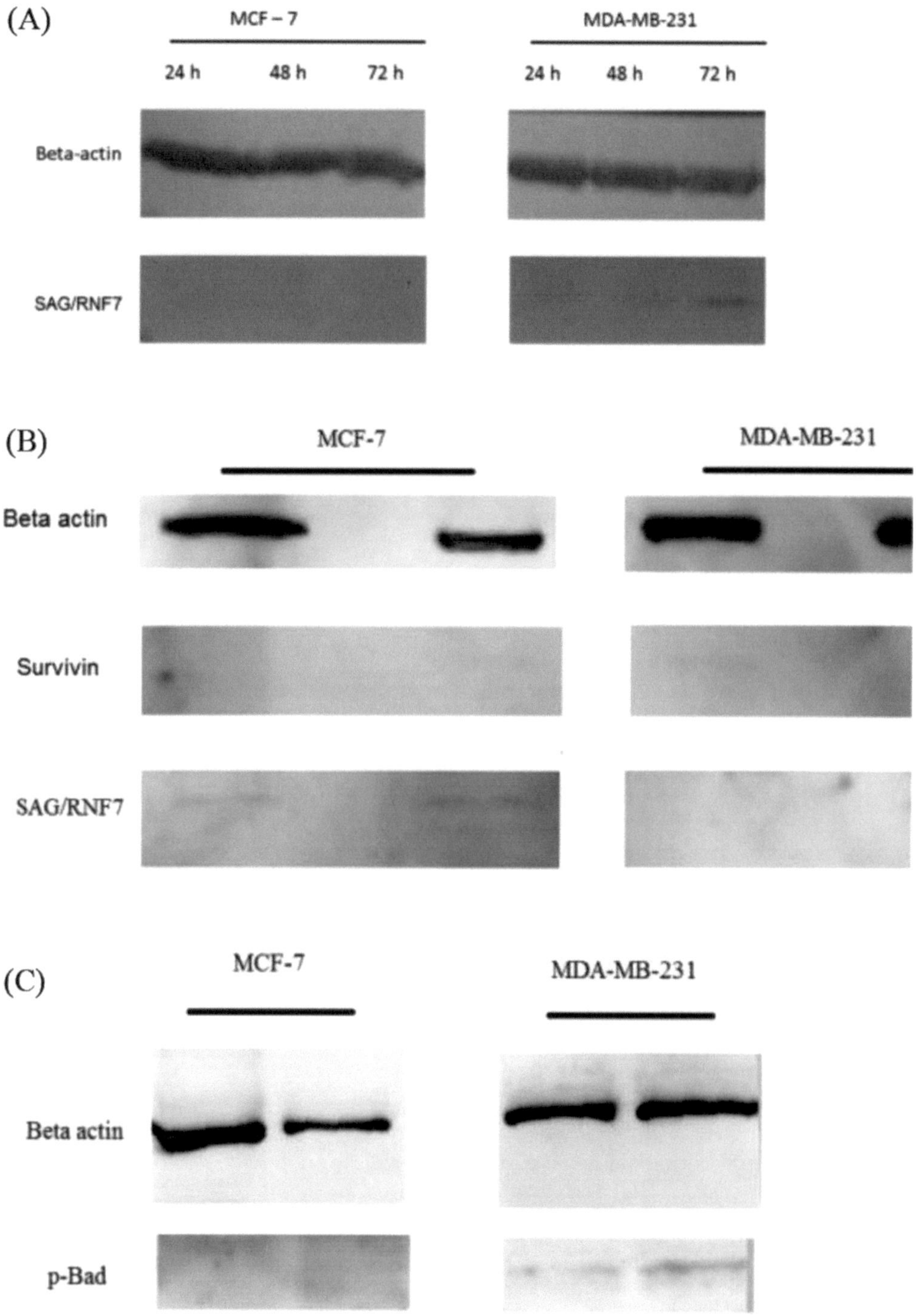

Figure 4. Western blot analysis of anti-apoptotic proteins (A) SAG at 24, 48 and 72 h, and (B) SAG and survivin after 48 h, together with (C) inactivated phosphorylated form of Bad. The data are representative of two independent experiments. Whole cell lysate was loaded as 40 μg proteins in each lane. β-actin was used as house-keeping control.

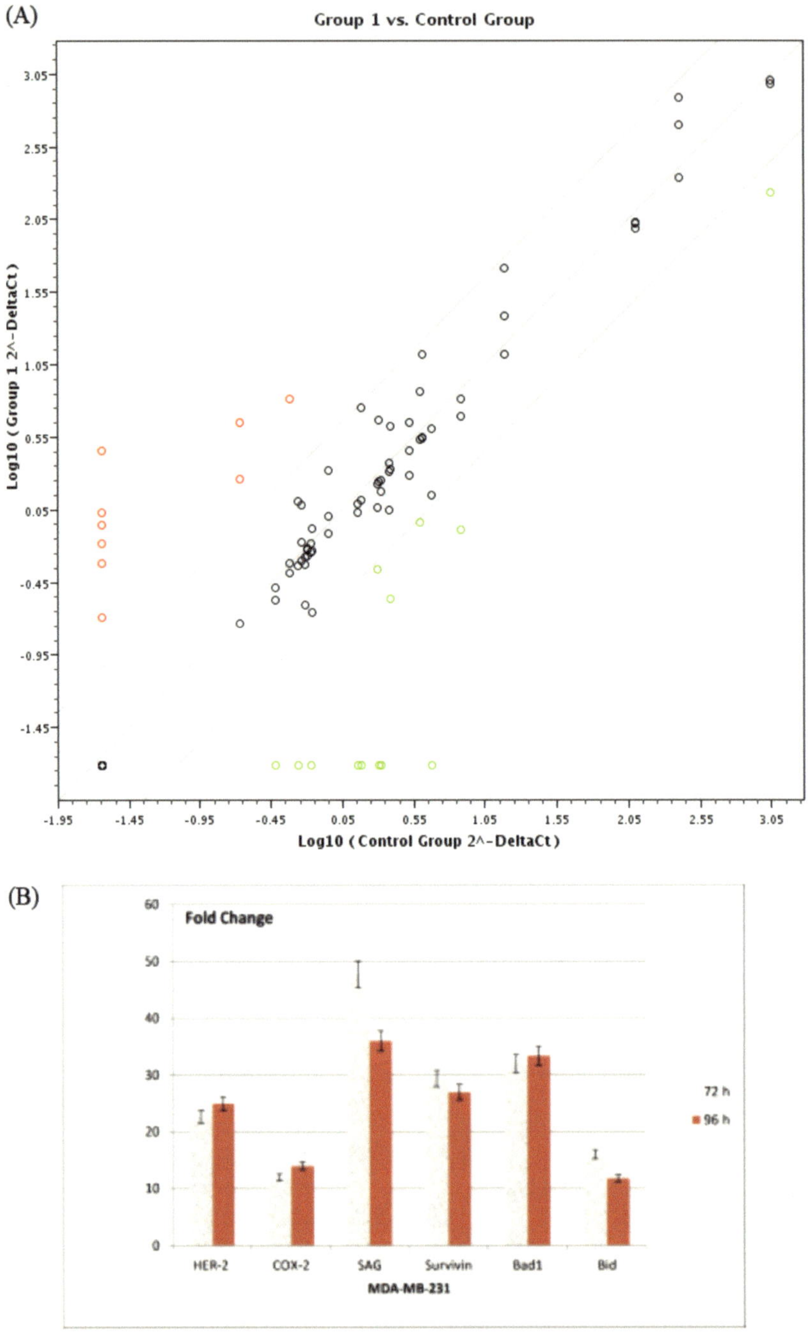

Figure 5. Effect of 100 μM etodolac addition on gene expressions of 6 genes chosen in relation to COX-2/apoptotic pathway after 72 and 96 h incubations. (A) Scattered plot analysis created by the software. The data points between the lines represent non-regulated proteins with insignificant fold-changes, where dots above the diagonals correspond to up- and dots below the diagonals correspond to down-regulations respectively. (B) Bar graph of fold changes observed in MDA-MB-231 cells. Regulations in MCF-7 cell line were minor, except negative regulation of BCL2L11, which correlated with positive regulations in Bak and Bax genes (data not shown).

5. Discussion

The expression of COX-1 and COX-2 in breast cell line cultures was studied in an early report by Liu et al. [41]. The data revealed that COX-2 is one of the markers showing differential expression between metastatic (MDA-MB-231) and non-metastatic hormone-responsive cell lines (MCF-7). Metastatic cell line had clearly high constitutive expression of COX-2 and a correlated increase in PGE2 levels. PGE2 production was firmly determined by phospholipase A2 availability, which is known to be high in metastatic MDA-MB-231 cell line, and COX2 activity, that is also shown to be higher in this cell line. These findings were further confirmed by a later study comparing COX-2 activity between colon cancer cell line HT-29 and its metastatic variant HT-29/Inv3 [40]. In prostate cancer cell lines, dose-response relation was found to be weaker for etodolac compared to NS-398, another selective COX-2 inhibitor [11]. Strange finding was that COX-2 expression did not necessarily correlated with its activity and etodolac was able to suppress PGE2 and tumour invasiveness without effecting protein COX-2 levels [14, 39]. Similarly, COX-2 expression and apoptosis were examined in HT-29 colon cancer cell lines, and high expression of COX-2 was detected in HT-29 cells with mutant APC. When full-length wild-type APC was expressed in the same line, the cell growth was declined and apoptosis was induced parallel to COX-2 down-regulation. However, activity tests showed that even though COX-2 expression exists, it is catalytically inactive in these cells [9].

Following these reports, the role of COX-2/PGE2 signalling in tumourigenesis, angiogenesis or suppression of apoptosis was further documented by many other studies and these fostered new therapeutic approaches based on various selective coxib derivatives. Clinical applications, however, demonstrated that the usage of NSAIDs or in particular coxibs as promoting anti-cancer agents has several drawbacks. Besides their serious side effects in gastrointestinal and cardiovascular systems, problems such as COX-2-independent anti-carcinogenic effects, or interferences with other eicosanoid pathways, signifies that great caution should be taken in the clinical use of these drugs [42]. Therefore, assessment of molecular changes in detail under different conditions could provide valuable foresight for future applications.

Although quite complex, carcinogenesis involves several main routes to follow in cell transformation. Limitless replicative capacity of cells could be a result of uncontrolled responses to growth signals, due to a constitutive receptor/ligand activity or insensitivity to growth signal inhibitors, cell cycle checkpoint defects, interfering with programmed cell death pathways, and sustained angiogenesis causing tumour invasion and metastasis.

Many signal transduction pathways cross talk and further complicate this picture. Studies focusing on cellular mechanisms of coxibs, in particular of etodolac and celecoxib, also reflect similar multi-facet picture.

In light of these observations, proteins playing substantial role in apoptotic fate were investigated to better understand the relations between COX-2/PGE2 and carcinogenesis. HER-2 (ERBB-2) and COX-2 were utilized to verify the already-identified correlation between high expression and invasiveness of the cells. As expected, MDA-MB-231 cells displayed higher expression levels of these genes and expressions were further up-regulated upon etodolac addition. Even though etodolac is a known Cox-2 inhibitor, as discussed above, its anti-proliferative effects may be

Cox-2 independent. A clinical study on breast cancers recently reported a significant increase in COX-2 gene expression levels upon etodolac addition, correlated with cyclin D1 reduction [43].

Etodolac induced an early increase in Bad gene expression, accompanied by Bax up-regulation and Bcl-2 down-regulation in MCF-7 cells, similar to the results previously reported for chemotherapeutic agents Taxol and Thiotepa [44]. Bad is able to regulate apoptosis by binding to the anti-apoptotic Bcl-2 family members Bcl-2 or Bcl-xL. This regulation proceeds post-translationally through modifications by kinases or phosphatases rather than transcriptional processes. Since only the unphosphorylated form of Bad is able to bind Bcl-xL or Bcl-2 to drive apoptotic process, we tested post-translational modifications through Western blot analyses. Phosphorylated form of the protein was enriched not in MCF-7 but in MDA-MB-231 cells. Phosphorylated form of Bad is inactive and explicitly induces growth and cancer development. The relation between protein levels and development or progression of different cancer types, including breast cancer, was recently examined both in cancer cell lines and on large-scale clinical data collected from The Moffitt Cancer Center Total Cancer Care repository [45]. Our results, in agreement with these findings, confirm the role of Bad in breast cancer cells and exhibit antagonistic action of etodolac in two cell lines with benign and malign characteristics. Bad phosphorylation would be one effective point in metastatic behaviour of MDA-MB-231 cell line. In addition to that, SAG and survivin were also clearly up-regulated in MDA-MB-231. Strangely, SAG increment was prominent in cells treated with 100 μM etodolac for 72 h.

SAG/ROC/Rbx/Hrt, also known as RNF7, is a member of zinc RING finger gene family, first characterized by Sun et al. [46]. This protein is a part of SCF E3 ubiquitin ligase complex and promotes polyubiquitination of various proteins involved in cell metabolism, signal transduction, cell cycle progression and apoptosis. Its reactive oxygen species (ROS)-scavenging activity protects cells from apoptosis induced by mitogenic factors such as ROS, hypoxia, stress, radiation, and so on and promotes cell survival. SAG levels were found to be higher in malignant cells and indicated as a potential prognostic marker at several cancer types [47, 48]. We found a reverse correlation of SAG, Bcl-xL and p53 expressions and overall survival of the advanced stage cervical carcinoma patients, as well as rectal cancer patients [49]. Apoptotic effects of SAG silencing were investigated in different cancer cell lines. Among the major pro-apoptotic proteins (Bax, Bak, Puma, Bim, Bad and NOXA) and anti-apoptotic proteins (Bcl-2, Mcl-1, survivin, XIAP, Bcl-xL and cIAP2), only NOXA was substantially regulated [50]. Therefore, in addition to known apoptotic markers, such as Bcl-2, Bax, Bak and Bad, we also wanted to examine if a potential association exists between SAG/NOXA- and COX-2/PGE2-related mechanisms leading to cell proliferation or apoptosis. As stated above, etodolac addition induced SAG up-regulation in both high-dose-short-time and low-dose-long-time applications in invasive cell line MDA-MB-231. NOXA expression was in basal levels, but there was no detectable down-regulation correlated with SAG levels.

In cancer, uncontrolled proliferation of cells leads to insufficient blood supply to the tissue, through the generation of aberrant microvessels. Lack of oxygen supply induces hypoxia-induced factor (HIF-1), which in turn activates SAG and SAG drives HIF-1α degradation through a feedback mechanism [51]. The role of hypoxia in the regulation of COX-2, on the other hand, was found to be an up-regulation of Cox-2 protein levels and correlated with hypoxia-inducible factor (HIF)-1α induction. A feedback loop, similar to SAG turnover, was reported in COX-2 pathway, in which COX-2/PGE2 up-regulation due to hypoxia enhances

http://dx.doi.org/10.5772/67855

HIF-1α transcriptional activity and this reinforces COX-2 up-regulation through a feedback mechanism [52, 53]. BNIP3 was another protein we tested in our panel. BNIP3 is known to be activated by hypoxia, and this activation results in enhanced mitochondrial membrane permeability and apoptosis [54, 55]. There was no definite change in neither HIF-1α nor BNIP3 levels (data not shown). In brief, among the sensitizers we tested (Bad, NOXA and BNIP3), only Bad was effectively regulated and etodolac does not show any straight regulation on hypoxia-related proteins. Our study marks the fact that in breast cancer, only the triple-negative invasive cell line was responsive to the effects of etodolac. MDA-MB-231 cell line promptly induced COX-2/HER2 expressions upon etodolac addition. HIF-1, BNIP3 and TP53 up-regulations in MDA-MB-231 were weak and these changes were reversing (down-regulation) for MCF-7 cells, but in similar levels. Up-regulation of anti-apoptotic proteins (SAG, survivin and Bcl-2) in MDA-MB-231 cell line was discernible in short times and became more evident when incubation time was extended to 3–4 days.

6. Conclusions

In this study, anti-proliferative and apoptotic effects of etodolac were investigated in breast cancer cell lines, MCF-7 and MDA-MB-231. Anti-proliferative and apoptotic changes were found to be pronounced only after high concentrations. Cox-2/HER2 over-expression was confirmed in invasive cell line MDA-MB-231. Regulation of mitochondrial Bcl-2 family proteins was moderate and pro- and anti-apoptotic proteins showed similar but reverse distributions. However, there was a prompt transcriptional up-regulation of Bad in MCF-7 and a slower response in MDA-MB-231 cells as the accumulation of phosphorylated form of Bad, suggesting a prominent role for Bad-mediated apoptotic pathway. In addition, SAG and survivin proteins increased in MDA-MB-231 cells in a dose-time-dependent manner. We believe that these findings would be supportive for future studies targeting etodolac-based therapies, as it reveals that apoptotic factors are differentially regulated in hormone-responsive and invasive cell lines.

Acknowledgements

This research is supported by the Scientific Research Project Commission of Marmara University (Project Number: SAG-A-080715-0313).

Author details

Oya Orun[1]*, Pınar Mega Tiber[1] and Sevgi Koçyiğit Sevinç[1,2]

*Address all correspondence to: oyaorun@yahoo.com

1 Biophysics Department, School of Medicine, Marmara University, Istanbul, Turkey

2 Biophysics Department, Faculty of Medicine, Dumlupinar University, Kütahya, Turkey

References

[1] Thun MJ, Henley SJ, Patrono C. Nonsteroidal anti-inflammatory drugs as anticancer agents: mechanistic, pharmacologic, and clinical issues. J Natl Cancer Inst. 2002;94(4):252-66.

[2] Chell S, Patsos HA, Qualtrough D, H-Zadeh AM, Hicks DJ, Kaidi A, et al. Prospects in NSAID-derived chemoprevention of colorectal cancer. Biochem Soc Trans. 2005; 33(4):667-71.

[3] Zimmermann KC, Sarbia M, Schrör K, Weber A-A. Constitutive cyclooxygenase-2 expression in healthy human and rabbit gastric mucosa. Mol Pharmacol. 1998;54(3): 536-40.

[4] Maślińska D, Kaliszek A, Opertowska J, Toborowicz J, Deregowski K, Szukiewicz D. Constitutive expression of cyclooxygenase-2 (COX-2) in developing brain. A. Choroid plexus in human fetuses. Folia Neuropathol. 1999;37(4):287-91.

[5] Kirkby NS, Chan MV, Zaiss AK, Garcia-Vaz E, Jiao J, Berglund LM, et al. Systematic study of constitutive cyclooxygenase-2 expression: Role of NF-κB and NFAT transcriptional pathways. Proc Natl Acad Sci. 2016;113(2):434-9.

[6] Lazzaroni M, Bianchi Porro G. Gastrointestinal side-effects of traditional non-steroidal anti-inflammatory drugs and new formulations. Aliment Pharmacol Ther. 2004;20(s2):48-58.

[7] Pawlosky N. Cardiovascular risk: Are all NSAIDs alike? Can Pharm J/Rev des Pharm du Canada. 2013;146(2):80-3.

[8] Kirkby NS, Zaiss AK, Urquhart P, Jiao J, Austin PJ, Al-Yamani M, et al. LC-MS/MS confirms that COX-1 drives vascular prostacyclin whilst gene expression pattern reveals non-vascular sites of COX-2 expression. PLoS One. 2013;8(7):e69524.

[9] Hsi LC, Joon Baek S, Eling TE. Lack of cyclooxygenase-2 activity in HT-29 human colorectal carcinoma cells. Exp Cell Res. 2000;256(2):563-70.

[10] Kobayashi M, Nakamura S, Shibata K, Sahara N, Shigeno K, Shinjo K, et al. Etodolac inhibits EBER expression and induces Bcl-2-regulated apoptosis in Burkitt's lymphoma cells. Eur J Haematol. 2005;75(3):212-20.

[11] Kamijo T, Sato T, Nagatomi Y, Kitamura T. Induction of apoptosis by cyclooxygenase-2 inhibitors in prostate cancer cell lines. Int J Urol. 2001;8(7):S35-9.

[12] Benoit V, Relic B, Leval X de, Chariot A, Merville M-P, Bours V. Regulation of HER-2 oncogene expression by cyclooxygenase-2 and prostaglandin E2. Oncogene. 2004;23(8):1631-5.

[13] Sandler AB, Dubinett SM. COX-2 inhibition and lung cancer. Semin Oncol. 2004;31(2 Suppl 7):45-52.

[14] Ferguson S, Hébert RL, Laneuville O. NS-398 upregulates constitutive cyclooxygenase-2 expression in the M-1 cortical collecting duct cell line. J Am Soc Nephrol. 1999;10(11):2261-71.

[15] Dogné J-M, Supuran CT, Pratico D. Adverse cardiovascular effects of the coxibs. J Med Chem. 2005;48(7):2251-7.

[16] Half E, Arber N. Colon cancer: preventive agents and the present status of chemoprevention. Expert Opin Pharmacother. 2009;10(2):211-9.

[17] Riendeau D, Percival MD, Boyce S, Brideau C, Charleson S, Cromlish W, et al. Biochemical and pharmacological profile of a tetrasubstituted furanone as a highly selective COX-2 inhibitor. Br J Pharmacol. 1997;121(1):105-17.

[18] Tacconelli S, Capone ML, Patrignani P. Clinical pharmacology of novel selective COX-2 inhibitors. Curr Pharm Des. 2004;10(6):589-601.

[19] Giuliano F, Ferraz JG, Pereira R, de Nucci G, Warner TD. Cyclooxygenase selectivity of non-steroid anti-inflammatory drugs in humans: ex vivo evaluation. Eur J Pharmacol. 2001;426(1-2):95-103.

[20] O'Callaghan G, Houston A. Prostaglandin E2 and the EP receptors in malignancy: possible therapeutic targets? Br J Pharmacol. 2015;172(22):5239-50.

[21] Sugimoto Y, Narumiya S. Prostaglandin E receptors. J Biol Chem. 2007; 282(16):11613-7.

[22] Bluwstein A, Kumar N, Léger K, Traenkle J, Oostrum J van, Rehrauer H, et al. PKC signaling prevents irradiation-induced apoptosis of primary human fibroblasts. Cell Death Dis. 2013;4(2):e498.

[23] Lee JL, Kim A, Kopelovich L, Bickers DR, Athar M. Differential expression of E prostanoid receptors in murine and human non-melanoma skin cancer. J Invest Dermatol. 2005;125(4):818-25.

[24] Tober KL, Wilgus TA, Kusewitt DF, Thomas-Ahner JM, Maruyama T, Oberyszyn TM. Importance of the EP1 receptor in cutaneous UVB-induced inflammation and tumor development. J Invest Dermatol. 2006;126(1):205-11.

[25] Chang H-H, Young SH, Sinnett-Smith J, Chou CEN, Moro A, Hertzer KM, et al. Prostaglandin E2 activates the mTORC1 pathway through an EP4/cAMP/PKA- and EP1/Ca2+-mediated mechanism in the human pancreatic carcinoma cell line PANC-1. Am J Physiol Cell Physiol. 2015;309(10):C639-49.

[26] Rundhaug JE, Simper MS, Surh I, Fischer SM. The role of the EP receptors for prostaglandin E2 in skin and skin cancer. Cancer Metastasis Rev. 2011;30(3-4):465-80.

[27] Amara SG, Kuhar MJ. Neurotransmitter transporters: recent progress. Annu Rev Neurosci. 1993;16:73-93.

[28] Shigemura K, Shirakawa T, Wada Y, Kamidono S, Fujisawa M, Gotoh A. Antitumor effects of etodolac, a selective cyclooxygenase-II inhibitor, against human prostate cancer cell lines in vitro and in vivo. Urology. 2005;66(6):1239-44.

[29] Shamas-Din A, Kale J, Leber B, Andrews DW. Mechanisms of action of Bcl-2 family proteins. Cold Spring Harb Perspect Biol. 2013;5(4):a008714-a008714.

[30] Lomonosova E, Chinnadurai G. BH3-only proteins in apoptosis and beyond: an overview. Oncogene. 2008;27(Suppl 1):S2-19.

[31] Czabotar PE, Lessene G, Strasser A, Adams JM. Control of apoptosis by the BCL-2 protein family: implications for physiology and therapy. Nat Rev Mol Cell Biol. 2013;15(1):49-63.

[32] Gallicchio M, Rosa a C, Dianzani C, Brucato L, Benetti E, Collino M, et al. Celecoxib decreases expression of the adhesion molecules ICAM-1 and VCAM-1 in a colon cancer cell line (HT29). Br J Pharmacol. 2008;153(5):870-8.

[33] Fatima N, Yi M, Ajaz S, Stephens RM, Stauffer S, Greenwald P, et al. Altered gene expression profiles define pathways in colorectal cancer cell lines affected by celecoxib. Cancer Epidemiol Biomarkers Prev. 2008;17(11):3051-61.

[34] Zhu J, Huang J-W, Tseng P-H, Yang Y-T, Fowble J, Shiau C-W, et al. From the cyclooxygenase-2 inhibitor celecoxib to a novel class of 3-phosphoinositide-dependent protein kinase-1 inhibitors. Cancer Res. 2004;64(12):4309-18.

[35] Kulp SK, Yang Y-T, Hung C-C, Chen K-F, Lai J-P, Tseng P-H, et al. 3-phosphoinositide-dependent protein kinase-1/Akt signaling represents a major cyclooxygenase-2-independent target for celecoxib in prostate cancer cells. Cancer Res. 2004;64(4):1444-51.

[36] Grosch S, Maier TJ, Schiffmann S, Geisslinger G. Cyclooxygenase-2 (COX-2)-independent anticarcinogenic effects of selective COX-2 inhibitors. J Natl Cancer Inst. 2006;98(11):736-47.

[37] Roy D, Arason G, Chowdhury B. Profiling of cell cycle genes of breast cells exposed to etodolac. Oncology Rep. 2010; 23: 1383-91.

[38] Küçükgüzel SG, Koç D, Çıkla-Süzgün P, Özsavcı D, Bingöl-Özakpınar Ö, Mega-Tiber P, et al. Synthesis of tolmetin hydrazide-hydrazones and discovery of a potent apoptosis inducer in colon cancer cells. Arch Pharm (Weinheim). 2015;348(10):730-42.

[39] Dai Z-J, Ma X-B, Kang H-F, Gao J, Min W-L, Guan H-T, et al. Antitumor activity of the selective cyclooxygenase-2 inhibitor, celecoxib, on breast cancer in Vitro and in Vivo. Cancer Cell Int. 2012;12(1):53.

[40] Chen WS, Wei SJ, Liu JM, Hsiao M, Kou-Lin J, Yang WK. Tumor invasiveness and liver metastasis of colon cancer cells correlated with cyclooxygenase-2 (COX-2) expression and inhibited by a COX-2-selective inhibitor, etodolac. Int J Cancer. 2001;91(6):894-9.

[41] Liu XH, Rose DP. Differential expression and regulation of cyclooxygenase-1 and -2 in two human breast cancer cell lines. Cancer Res. 1996;56(22):5125-7.

[42] Rigas B, Kashfi K. Cancer prevention: a new era beyond cyclooxygenase-2. J Pharmacol Exp Ther. 2005;314(1):1-8.

[43] Schwab RB, Kato S, Crain B, Pu M, Messer K, Weidner N, et al. A window-of-opportunity biomarker study of etodolac in resectable breast cancer. Cancer Med. 2015;4(10):1583-8.

[44] Tudor G, Aguilera A, Halverson DO, Laing ND, Sausville EA. Susceptibility to drug-induced apoptosis correlates with differential modulation of Bad, Bcl-2 and Bcl-xL protein levels. Cell Death Differ. 2000;7(6):574-86.

[45] Stickles XB, Marchion DC, Bicaku E, Al Sawah E, Abbasi F, Xiong Y, et al. BAD-mediated apoptotic pathway is associated with human cancer development. Int J Mol Med. 2015;35(4):1081-7.

[46] Sun Y, Tan M, Duan H, Swaroop M. *SAG/ROC/Rbx/Hrt*, a zinc RING finger gene family: molecular cloning, biochemical properties, and biological functions. Antioxid Redox Signal. 2001;3(4):635-50.

[47] Sasaki H, Yukiue H, Kobayashi Y, Moriyama S, Nakashima Y, Kaji M, et al. Expression of the sensitive to apoptosis gene, SAG, as a prognostic marker in nonsmall cell lung cancer. Int J Cancer. 2001;95(6):375-7.

[48] Ozden SA, Ozyurt H, Ozgen Z, Kilinc O, Oncel M, Gul AE, et al. Prognostic role of sensitive-to-apoptosis gene expression in rectal cancer. World J Gastroenterol. 2011; 17(44):4905-10.

[49] Orun O, Mega Tiber P, Baloglu L, Ozden S, Ozgen Z, Ozyurt H, et al. The association of apoptotic protein expressions sensitive to apoptosis gene, p73 and p53 with the prognosis of cervical carcinoma. Onco Targets Ther. 2014;7:2161-8.

[50] Jia L, Yang J, Hao X, Zheng M, He H, Xiong X, et al. Validation of SAG/RBX2/ROC2 E3 ubiquitin ligase as an anticancer and radiosensitizing target. Clin Cancer Res. 2010;16(3):814-24.

[51] Tan M, Gu Q, He H, Pamarthy D, Semenza GL, Sun Y. SAG/ROC2/RBX2 is a HIF-1 target gene that promotes HIF-1α ubiquitination and degradation. Oncogene. 2008;27 (10):1404-11.

[52] Jung Y-J, Isaacs JS, Lee S, Trepel J, Neckers L. IL-1 mediated up-regulation of HIF-1 via an NFkB/COX-2 pathway identifies HIF-1 as a critical link between inflammation and oncogenesis. FASEB J. 2003;17(14):2115-7.

[53] Zhong H, Willard M, Simons J. NS398 reduces hypoxia-inducible factor(HIF)-1α and HIF-1 activity: Multiple-level effects involving cyclooxygenase-2 dependent and independent mechanisms. Int J Cancer. 2004;112(4):585-95.

[54] Kubasiak LA, Hernandez OM, Bishopric NH, Webster KA. Hypoxia and acidosis activate cardiac myocyte death through the Bcl-2 family protein BNIP3. Proc Natl Acad Sci U S A. 2002;99(20):12825-30.

[55] Graham RM, Thompson JW, Webster KA. BNIP3 promotes calcium and calpain-dependent cell death. Life Sci. 2015;142:26-35.